Herbal Remedies

ALTERNATIVE THERAPIES

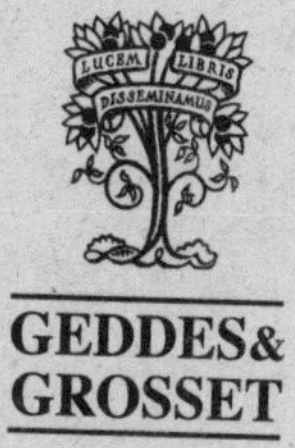

GEDDES & GROSSET

Published 2007 by Geddes & Grosset,
David Dale House, New Lanark ML11 9DJ, Scotland

Cover photograph courtesy of Brooks & Brown/Science Photo Library

First published 1996
Reprinted 1999 (twice), 2001, 2007

ISBN 978 1 85534 224 8

Printed and bound in India

Contents

Warning: Do not undertake any course of treatment without the advice of your doctor.

A-Z of Herbal Remedies

Aconite *Aconitum napellus.*
COMMON NAME: monkshood, blue rocket, friar's cap, wolfsbane.
OCCURRENCE: indigenous to mountain slopes in the Alps and Pyrenees. Introduced into England very early, before 900 AD.
PARTS USED: the leaves used fresh and the root when dried. It contains alkaloidal material—aconitine, benzaconine and aconine amongst other compounds.
MEDICINAL USES: the plant is poisonous and should not be used except under medical advice. It is an anodyne, febrifuge and sedative. Used for reducing fever and inflammation in the treatment of catarrh, tonsillitis and croup. It may be used in controlling heart spasm.
ADMINISTERED AS: tincture, liniment and occasionally as injection.

Agrimony *Agrimonia eupatoria.*
COMMON NAME: church steeples, cockleburr, sticklewort.
OCCURRENCE: field borders, ditches and hedges throughout England. Found locally in Scotland.
PARTS USED: the herb. Contains a particular volatile oil, tannin and a bitter principle.
MEDICINAL USES: mild astringent, tonic, diuretic, deobstruent. It has a reputation for curing liver complaints and is very good for skin eruptions and blood diseases. Also recommended to treat the sting and bite of snakes.
ADMINISTERED AS: liquid extract.

Alder *Alnus glutinosa.*
COMMON NAME: betula alnus.
OCCURRENCE: commonly found throughout Britain, usually in moist woods or by streams.
PARTS USED: the bark, wood, shoots, catkins and leaves have all been used as dyes. The bark and leaves contain tannic acid.
MEDICINAL USES: tonic and astringent. Used as a decoction to bathe swelling and inflammation, particularly of the throat.
ADMINISTERED AS: decoction.

Aloes *Aloe perryi, Aloe vera.*
OCCURRENCE: indigenous to East and South Africa and introduced into the West Indies.
PARTS USED: the drug aloes is described as the liquid evaporated to dryness which drains from the leaves. It contains two aloin compounds, barbaloin and isobarbaloin, as well as amorphous aloin, resin and aloe-emodin in differing proportions.
MEDICINAL USES: emmenagogue, purgative, vermifuge, anthelmintic. It is generally administered along with carminative and anodyne drugs, and acts on the lower bowel. The liquid form may be used externally to ease skin irritation.
ADMINISTERED AS: fluid extract, powdered extract, decoction, tincture.

Allspice *Pimento officinalis.*
COMMON NAME: pimento, Jamaica pepper, clove pepper.
OCCURRENCE: indigenous to the West Indies and South America; cultivated in Jamaica and central America.
PARTS USED: the fruit, which contains a volatile oil made up of eugenol, a sesquiterpene and other unknown chemicals.
MEDICINAL USES: aromatic, stimulant, carminative. Allspice acts on the gastro-intestinal tract and is usually added to drinks tonics and

purgatives for flavouring. The spice may also be used for flatulent indigestion and hysteria. Allspice is frequently used as a spice and condiment in food or drinks.
ADMINISTERED AS: essential oil, distilled water, powdered fruit, fluid extract.

Almond, Sweet *Amygdalus communis* var. *dulais*. **Almond, Bitter** *Amygdalus commis* var. *amara*.
OCCURRENCE: native trees of western Asia and North Africa and cultivated in most Mediterranean countries and Great Britain.
PARTS USED: the nut and the oil expressed from it.
MEDICINAL USES: sweet almonds have demulcent and nutritive properties, but since the outer skin can cause irritation of the alimentary canal, almonds are normally blanched and the skin removed before being used as food. The oil produced is emollient, demulcent, nutritive and slightly laxative, and is mainly used in cosmetics but is also taken internally as a medicine. It is of benefit in allaying acrid juices, softening and relaxing solid materials, bronchial diseases, tickling coughs, hoarseness and nephritic pains. Sweet almonds are made into emulsions with barley water or gum arabic to treat gravel, stone, kidney disorders and bladder and biliary duct problems, with more success than almond oil.

Bitter almonds yield a volatile oil upon distillation with water which is used as a flavouring agent. These almonds contain the glucoside amygdalin and the chemical emulsin that acts on the glucoside to produce glucose, prussic acid and benzaldehyde in the presence of water. Prussic acid is poisonous and use of bitter almond oil must be carefully monitored. In the Middle Ages, the oil was used for intermittent fevers, hydrophobia and as an aperient, diuretic and vermifuge drug, but it is seldom administered medicinally now. The cake left after expressing the oil has a special dietary value and is often

made into flour for cakes and biscuits for diabetic patients. Almond oil is used in trade as a lubricant for watches, and in soaps and toiletries.
ADMINISTERED AS: expressed oil, bitter almond oil (with prussic acid removed).

Anemone, Wood *Anemone nemorosa.*
COMMON NAME: crowfoot, windflower, smell fox.
OCCURRENCE: found in woods and thickets across Great Britain.
PARTS USED: the root, leaves and juice.
MEDICINAL USES: this species of plant is much less widely used than it has been previously. It used to be good for leprosy, lethargy, eye inflammation and headaches. An ointment made of the leaves is said to be effective in cleansing malignant ulcers.
ADMINISTERED AS: decoction, fresh leaves and root, ointment.

Anemone, Pulsatilla *Anemone pulsatilla.*
COMMON NAME: pasqueflower, meadow anemone, wind flower.
OCCURRENCE: found locally in chalk downs and limestone areas of England.
PARTS USED: the whole herb. It produces oil of anemone upon distillation with water.
MEDICINAL USES: nervine, antispasmodic, alterative and diaphoretic. It is beneficial in disorders of mucous membranes and of the respiratory and digestive passages. Can be used to treat asthma, whooping cough and bronchitis.
ADMINISTERED AS: fluid extract.

Angelica *Angelica archangelica.*
COMMON NAME: garden angelica, *Archangelica officinalis.*
OCCURRENCE: found native to some sites in Scotland although more abundant in Lapland and is a common garden plant in England.

PARTS USED: the root, leaves and seeds. The leaves contain volatile oil, valeric acid, angelic acid, a bitter principle and a resin called angelicin. The roots contain terebangelene and other terpenes while the seeds also yield two acid compounds.
MEDICINAL USES: angelica has carminative, stimulant, diaphoretic, diuretic, aromatic, stomachic, tonic and expectorant properties and is good for colds, coughs, pleurisy, wind, colic and rheumatism. It is used as a stimulating expectorant and is good for digestion.
ADMINISTERED AS: powdered root, liquid extract, infusion or as a poultice.

Angostura *Galipea officinalis.*
COMMON NAME: cusparia bark, *Cusparia febrifuga, Bonplandia trifoliata, Galipea cusparia.*
OCCURRENCE: a small tree native to tropical South America.
PARTS USED: the dried bark, which has the active ingredients angosturin, the alkaloids galipine, cusparine, galipidine, cusparidine and cuspareine, as well as a volatile oil and an unidentified glucoside.
MEDICINAL USES: aromatic, bitter, tonic, stimulant, purgative. There is a long history of usage by native South Americans as a stimulant tonic. It is useful in bilious diarrhoea and dysentery, but in large doses it has a purgative and cathartic effect on the body.
ADMINISTERED AS: infusion, powdered bark, tincture, fluid extract.

Anise *Pimpinella anisum.*
COMMON NAME: aniseed.
OCCURRENCE: native to Egypt, Greece, Crete and western Asia, its cultivation spread to central Europe and North Africa.
PARTS USED: the fruit. Upon distillation, the fruit yields a fragrant

volatile oil that is made up of anethol, choline, a fixed oil, sugar and mucilage.
MEDICINAL USES: carminative and pectoral. It is very useful against coughs and chest infections and is made into lozenges or smoked to clear the chest. Aniseed tea is good for infant catarrh, and aids digestion in adults. Anise seed is an ingredient of cathartic and aperient pills, to relieve flatulence and lessen the griping caused by purgative herbs. It can also be given in convulsions quite safely.
ADMINISTERED AS: essence, essential oil, tincture, powdered seeds, tea and pills.

Apple *Pyrus malus*.
COMMON NAME: wild apple, *Malus communis*, crab-tree.
OCCURRENCE: native to Great Britain and found throughout the temperate regions of the northern hemisphere.
PARTS USED: the fruit and bark. Apples contain water, protein material, carbonaceous matter, vitamins, organic acids, salts of potassium, sodium, carbon and magnesium.
MEDICINAL USES: diuretic, slightly astringent. The organic acids in the fruit benefit sedentary people and ease liver problems, gout and indigestion. Apple juice or cider is drunk frequently in some areas e.g. Normandy, where problems of stone or calculus are unknown because of the diuretic effects of apples. Apples can also help cure constipation, scurvy, sleeplessness or bilious complaints. They act as an excellent dentifrice (tooth cleanser) and are applied as a poultice to sore eyes when rotten. A decoction of the bark is used against intermittent and bilious fevers, while cooked apples are used in sore throats, eye problems, and in skin and tissue infected with the *Streptococcus pyogenes* bacterium. Dropsy is helped by drinking cider in which horseradish was steeped.

ADMINISTERED AS: fresh fruit, expressed juice, fermented drink, infusion, decoction, poultice.

Apricot *Prunus armeniaca.*
COMMON NAME: apricock, *Armeniaca vulgaris.*
OCCURRENCE: originally found in northern China, the Himalaya region and temperate Asia. Now cultivated across temperate regions of Europe. Introduced into England in the sixteenth century.
PARTS USED: the kernels and the oil expressed from them. The oil contains olein and the glyceride of linolic acid. The cake left after oil removal produces an essential oil upon distillation that contains the glucoside amygdalin and is chemically identical to the essential oil from the almond. It is used in confectionery and as a food flavouring.
MEDICINAL USES: apricot oil is substituted for oil of almonds in cosmetics, because of its lower cost. It has a softening action on the skin.
ADMINISTERED AS: expressed oil, essential oil.

Areca Nut *Areca catechu.*
COMMON NAME: betel nut, pinang.
OCCURRENCE: a tree cultivated in the East Indies, India and Sri Lanka.
PARTS USED: the seeds contain a large amount of tannin, gallic acid, a fixed oil, lignin and a volatile oil. They also contain three alkaloids, arcoline, arecain and guracine with the second listed being the active principle.
MEDICINAL USES: aromatic, astringent, taenacide and mydriatic. The native people chew these nuts, which stain the teeth, lips and excrement red. Taken internally, the seeds expel tapeworms and cause contraction of the pupil of the eye. Areca nut is also made into a toothpaste in Britain.
ADMINISTERED AS: powdered nut, fluid extract.

Arnica *Arnica montana.*
COMMON NAME: mountain tobacco, leopard's bane.
OCCURRENCE: indigenous to central Europe but found in England and southern Scotland.
PARTS USED: the rhizome and flowers. They contain arnicin, tannin, phullin and a volatile oil.
MEDICINAL USES: stimulant, vulnerary and diuretic. It is used in external application to bruises and sprains but is rarely used internally as it irritates the stomach, and may cause severe poisoning. A tincture of arnica has been used to treat epilepsy and seasickness.
ADMINISTERED AS: tincture, poultice.

Arrach *Chenopodium olidum.*
COMMON NAME: stinking motherwort/arrach/goosefoot, dog's arrach, goat's arrach, netchweed.
OCCURRENCE: an annual herb found on waste ground or roadsides throughout Great Britain.
PARTS USED: herb. Contains trimethylamine, osmazome and nitrate of potash.
MEDICINAL USES: nervine, emmenagogue, anti-spasmodic. This is used in female hysteria and was formerly said to cure barrenness.
ADMINISTERED AS: an infusion, fluid extract or injection.

Arrowroot *Maranta arundinacea.*
COMMON NAME: *Maranta indica, M. ramosissima*, maranta starch or arrowroot, araruta, Bermuda arrowroot, Indian arrowroot.
OCCURRENCE: indigenous to the West Indies and central America. It is cultivated in Bengal, Java, the Philippines, Mauritius and West Africa.
PARTS USED: the dried, powdered starch from the rhizome.
MEDICINAL USES: nutritive, demulcent, non-irritating. Well suited

for infants and convalescents, particularly after bowel complaints. The jelly made of water or milk may be flavoured with sugar, lemon juice or fruit. The fresh rhizomes are mashed and applied to wounds from poisoned arrows, scorpion or spider bites and to stop gangrene. The freshly expressed juice of the rhizome, when mixed with water, is said to be a good antidote against vegetable poisons.
ADMINISTERED AS: fresh root, expressed juice, dietary item.

Asarabacca *Asarum europaeum.*
COMMON NAME: hazelwort, wild nard.
OCCURRENCE: asarabacca is the only British species of the birthwort family and is very rare. It is found in woodlands.
PARTS USED: the root and herb.
MEDICINAL USES: stimulant, tonic, emetic, purgative, aromatic and sternulatory. As dried powdered leaves of the herb, it is used in the preparation of snuffs, causing sneezing and giving relief to headaches and weak eyes. It has been utilized to remove mucus from the respiratory passages and may be an antidote to the bite of venomous snakes. The herb was formerly used as an emetic or purgative but its use has been replaced by safer drugs.
ADMINISTERED AS: tincture, emulsion.

Asparagus *Asparagus officinalis.*
COMMON NAME: sparrow grass.
OCCURRENCE: a rare native in Britain, but found wild on the southwest coast of England. It is cultivated as a food crop in parts of Scotland.
PARTS USED: the root.
MEDICINAL USES: this plant has diuretic, laxative, cardiac and sedative effects. It is recommended in cases of dropsy.
ADMINISTERED AS: expressed juice, decoction or made in a syrup.

Avens *Geum urbanum.*
COMMON NAME: colewort, herb bennet, city Avens, wild rue, way bennet, goldy star, clove root.
OCCURRENCE: a common hedgerow plant in Britain and Europe.
PARTS USED: the herb and root. The herb contains a volatile oil composed of eugenol and a glucoside, while the root also contains tannin.
MEDICINAL USES: an astringent, styptic, febrifuge, sudorific, stomachic, antiseptic, tonic and aromatic. It is useful in diarrhoea, sore throat, chills, fevers and headache amongst other complaints. An infusion may be used for skin problems, as a wash.
ADMINISTERED AS: an infusion, decoction or tincture.

Balm *Melissa officinalis.*
COMMON NAME: sweet balm, lemon balm, honey plant, cure-all.
OCCURRENCE: a common garden plant in Great Britain, which was naturalized into southern England at a very early period.
PARTS USED: the herb.
MEDICINAL USES: as a carminative, diaphoretic, or febrifuge. It can be made into a cooling tea for fever patients and balm is often used in combination with other herbs to treat colds and fever.
ADMINISTERED AS: an infusion.

Balmony *Chelone glabra.*
COMMON NAME: chelone, bitter herb, snake head, shellflower, turtlehead, turtle bloom, salt-rheum weed, glatte, the humming-bird tree, white chelone.
OCCURRENCE: it grows in swamps, wet woods and rivers in the eastern United States and Canada.
PARTS USED: the whole herb.

MEDICINAL USES: the fresh leaves are anti-bilious, anthelmintic, tonic and detergent in action and are used against consumption, dyspepsia, debility and jaundice. It has a peculiar action on the liver and diseases of that organ, while it is also effective in removing worms from children. When made into an ointment, balmony is recommended for inflamed tumours, ulcers, inflamed breasts and piles.
ADMINISTERED AS: a decoction, powdered herb, fluid extract, tincture.

Balsam of Peru *Myroxylon pereirae.*
COMMON NAME: Peruvian balsam, *Toluifera pereira*, *Myrosperum pereira.*
OCCURRENCE: this comes from a large tree that grows in the forest of El Salvador, central America.
PARTS USED: the balsam is an oleoresinous liquid that exudes from the tree after the bark has been beaten and scorched. It is soaked from the tree and boiled in water.
MEDICINAL USES: stimulant, expectorant, parasiticide. It is used in scabies, irritant skin diseases and acute eczema. The balsam is good in all chronic mucous afflictions, catarrh, leucorrhoea, diarrhoea and dysentery. It stimulates the heart and raises blood pressure. The liquid may be applied to sore nipples and discharges from the ear to effect healing.
ADMINISTERED AS: liquid form.

Baneberry *Actaea spicata.*
COMMON NAME: herb Christopher, bugbane, toadroot.
OCCURRENCE: a rare plant in Britain, found only in limestone districts of the Lake District and Yorkshire.
PARTS USED: the root.
MEDICINAL USES: antispasmodic. The plant is acrid and poisonous.

The root is used as a remedy for catarrh and some nervous disorders, but the plant must be used with great caution.
ADMINISTERED AS: infusion, dried or fresh root.

Barberry *Berberis vulgaris.*
COMMON NAME: berbery, pipperidge bush, *Berberis dumetorum.*
OCCURRENCE: a common bush that grows wild in some parts of England but is unlikely to be native to Scotland and Ireland.
PARTS USED: the root, root-bark and berries. The bark contains berberine, a bitter alkaloid, along with several other compounds.
MEDICINAL USES: as a tonic, purgative and antiseptic. It is normally used to treat jaundice and liver complaints, and is an aid to regulating digestion and stopping constipation. The berries are used to produce an acid drink that helps ease diarrhoea and fevers.
ADMINISTERED AS: powdered bark, fluid extract and solid extract.

Barley *Hordeum distichon* and *Hordeum vulgare.*
COMMON NAME: pearl barley, *Perlatum.*
OCCURRENCE: throughout Britain.
PARTS USED: decorticated seeds composed of eighty per cent starch and six per cent proteins, cellulose, etc.
MEDICINAL USES: barley is used to prepare a nutritive and demulcent drink for ill and fevered patients. Barley water is given to sick children suffering from diarrhoea or bowel inflammation etc. Malt extract is also used medicinally.
ADMINISTERED AS: an infusion and beverage.

Basil *Ocimum basilicum.*
COMMON NAME: sweet basil, garden basil.
OCCURRENCE: as a garden plant throughout Britain.
PARTS USED: the herb, which contains a volatile, camphoraceous oil.

MEDICINAL USES: aromatic with carminative and cooling properties. It is used to treat mild nervous disorders, and an infusion of basil is said to be good for obstructions of the internal organs and in stopping vomiting and nausea.
ADMINISTERED AS: a flavouring in food, dried leaves or an infusion.

Bayberry *Myrica corifera.*
COMMON NAME: candleberry, waxberry, tallow shrub, wax myrtle.
OCCURRENCE: widely distributed through America, Europe and Great Britain.
PARTS USED: the bark, which contains volatile oil, starch, lignin, tannic and gallic acids along with lesser compounds.
MEDICINAL USES: a powerful stimulant, astringent and tonic. The powdered bark may be used in poultices, often together with elm. A decoction is used to treat the throat and sore gums.
ADMINISTERED AS: an infusion, decoction, powder and injection.

Bearberry *Archostaphylos uva-ursi.*
COMMON NAME: *Arbutus uva-ursi, uva-ursi.*
OCCURRENCE: on heaths of the Scottish Highlands, south to Yorkshire, and in high mountains of Europe, Asia and America.
PARTS USED: the leaves, which contain arbutin as the chief constituent.
MEDICINAL USES: when made into an infusion, the leaves have a soothing, astringent and diuretic effect. This is of benefit in diseases affecting the bladder, and the kidneys, e.g. urethritis, cystitis, etc.
ADMINISTERED AS: an infusion.

Beech *Fagus Sylvatica.*
COMMON NAME: buche, boke, faggio, fagos.

OCCURRENCE: found in Europe, including Britain, although only indigenous to England.
PARTS USED: the oil of beech nuts, and beech tar.
MEDICINAL USES: beech tar is stimulating and antiseptic so is used internally as a stimulating expectorant to treat chronic bronchitis. It is used externally applied to various skin diseases.
ADMINISTERED AS: beech oil or beech tar.

Beetroot *Beta vulgaris.*
COMMON NAME: spinach beet, sea beet, garden beet, whit beet, mangel-wurzel.
OCCURRENCE: *Beta vulgaris* is native to southern Europe and is derived from the sea beet, *Beta maritima* which grows wild on the coasts of Europe, England, North Africa and Asia. There are many cultivated forms and varieties of beetroot with similar properties.
PARTS USED: the leaves and root. The root contains a pure fruit sugar which is easily taken up by the body, as well as starch and gum.
MEDICINAL USES: the juice of the white beet was said to be of a "cleansing, digestive quality" to "open up obstructions of the liver and spleen" and ease headaches. Beetroot is used to produce refined sugar, as a vegetable and to make wine or ale.
ADMINISTERED AS: dietary item, decoction, expressed juice.

Belladonna *Atropa belladonna.*
COMMON NAME: deadly nightshade, devil's cherries, dwale, black cherry, devil's herb, great morel.
OCCURRENCE: native to central and southern Europe but commonly grows in England.
PARTS USED: the roots and leaves. The root contains several alkaloid compounds, including hyoscyamine, atropine and

belladonnine. The same alkaloids are present in the leaves but the amount of each compound varies according to plant type and methods of storing and drying leaves.

MEDICINAL USES: as a narcotic, diuretic, sedative, mydriatic, antispasmodic. The drug is used as an anodyne in febrile conditions, night sweats and coughs. It is valuable in treating eye diseases and is used as a pain-relieving lotion to treat neuralgia, gout, rheumatism and sciatica. Belladonna is an extremely poisonous plant and should always be used under medical supervision. Cases of accidental poisoning and death are well-known. Despite this, it is a valuable drug used to treat a wide range of diseases.

ADMINISTERED AS: a liquid extract that is used to produce alcoholic extracts, plasters, liniment, suppositories, tincture and ointment.

Bergamot *Monarda didyma.*

COMMON NAME: scarlet monarda, Oswego tea, bee balm.

OCCURRENCE: a plant which is indigenous to North America.

PARTS USED: the oil extracted from the whole plant, and the leaves.

MEDICINAL USES: used in a similar manner to other plants containing thymol as an active chemical. Oil of bergamot has antiseptic, aromatic, carminative, tonic and antispasmodic properties. An infusion of the young leaves was a common beverage in the USA before tea became more common. The infusion is also good for coughs, sore throats, fevers and colds.

ADMINISTERED AS: essential oil, infusion, fluid extract.

Bethroot *Trillium pendulum, Trillium erectum.*

COMMON NAME: Indian shamrock, birthroot, lamb's quarters, wake-robin, Indian balm, ground lily.

OCCURRENCE: a native North American plant found in the western

and middle United States.
PARTS USED: the dried root and rhizome; the leaves.
MEDICINAL USES: antiseptic, astringent, tonic, expectorant, pectoral and alterative. It is useful in all cases of internal bleeding, profuse menstruation and pulmonary complaints. It is used to promote safe childbirth and delivery. The leaves may be applied to ulcers and tumours while the root makes a good antiseptic poultice to stop gangrene spreading or for skin diseases. It was used by the native Americans as a medicine.
ADMINISTERED AS: the powdered root, fresh leaves and infusion.

Betony, Wood *Stachys bentonica, Betonica officinalis.*
COMMON NAME: bishopswort.
OCCURRENCE: found wild in woodlands, or on heath or moorland but less common in Scotland.
PARTS USED: the herb.
MEDICINAL USES: aromatic, astringent and alterative. Betony was thought to be one of the best treatments for headaches and hangovers. It is normally combined with other herbs to produce a tonic for nervous affections, dyspepsia and rheumatism. The dried herb was also used to make a tea substitute and was smoked as tobacco.
ADMINISTERED AS: an infusion.

Bindweed, Greater *Convolvulus sepium.*
COMMON NAME: hedge convolvulus, old man's night cap, hooded bindweed, bearbind.
OCCURRENCE: a native of Britain which is abundant in England but rarer in Scotland.
PARTS USED: the resin produced from the roots.
MEDICINAL USES: the resin is normally made into a tincture. This preparation is then applied internally and has a purgative effect.

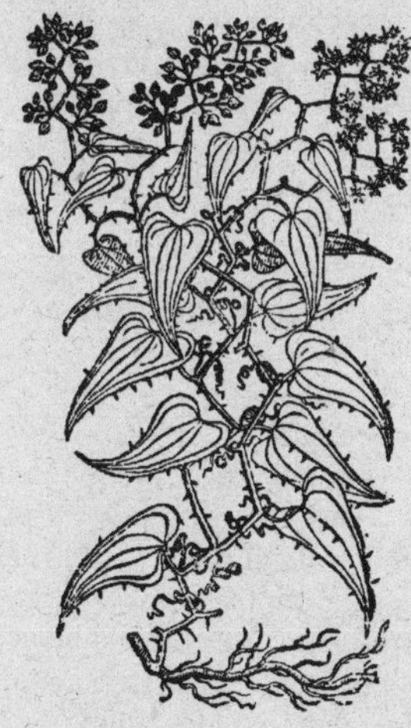
bindweed

The effects are not as pronounced as in the related plant species *Convulvus jalapa* (jalap bindweed) and *Convulvus scammonia* (Syrian bindweed).
ADMINISTERED AS: tincture.

Birch, Common *Betula alba.*
COMMON NAME: white birch, bouleau, berke, bereza.
OCCURRENCE: common in Europe, from Sicily to Iceland and also found in northern Asia.
PARTS USED: the bark and leaves. The bark contains tannic acid, behilin and behils camphor while the leaves contain betulorentic acid.
MEDICINAL USES: bitter and astringent. The bark yields oil of birch tar upon destructive distillation, which is very similar to oil of WINTERGREEN. The oil is used in skin disease ointments, e.g. treating eczema while it is also used as a component of insect repellent. Birch tea made of the leaves is recommended for gout, rheumatism and dropsy and is also said to be good for breaking up kidney stones. Sap from the tree is used to produce beer, wine, spirits and vinegar in various parts of Europe.
ADMINISTERED AS: oil, infusion.

Birthwort *Aristolochia longa.*
COMMON NAME: long-rooted birthwort.
OCCURRENCE: throughout Europe and Great Britain.

Bistort

PARTS USED: the root, which contains aristolochine.
MEDICINAL USES: aromatic and stimulant. It is useful in treating gout and rheumatism and may be used to clear obstructions after childbirth.
ADMINISTERED AS: powdered root.

Bistort *Polygonum bisorta.*
COMMON NAME: snakeweed, adderwort, twice writhen, osterick, Easter marigiant, English sepentary.
OCCURRENCE: a native of many parts of northern Europe, common in the north of England and southern Scotland.
PARTS USED: the root-stock which contains tannin, starch, gallic acid and gum.
MEDICINAL USES: a strong astringent and is mainly used in external and internal bleeding and haemorrhages from the lungs or stomach. Can be used to treat diarrhoea, dysentery, cholera and bowel complaints. Bistort is important in alleviating diabetes and as a mouth wash or gargle to "fasten loose teeth" and heal gum problems.
ADMINISTERED AS: a powder, fluid extract, decoction or injection.

Bitter root *Apocynum androsaemifolium.*
COMMON NAME: milkweed, dogsbane, fly-trap, wild cotton.
OCCURRENCE: found in mountainous regions of Europe and North America.
PARTS USED: the dried rhizome and roots. The active chemicals in the plant are a bitter principle called cymarin, and to a lesser extent the glucoside apocynamarin.
MEDICINAL USES: cardiac tonic, hydragogue, alterative. Bitter root is similar to foxglove in action and is very powerful in slowing the pulse and it also has a strong action on the vaso-motor system. It may irritate the mucous membranes, causing nausea and

purging of the bowels, so that it cannot be tolerated by all people. As a powerful hydrogogue it is good against fluid accumulation in the abdomen (ascites), particularly when it is linked to liver cirrhosis. It is also highly effective in treating dropsy which is related to heart failure. The plant's alterative powers are used against syphilis, scrofula and rheumatism. Because of irregular absorption of the drug through the gastro-intestinal tract, great care must be taken with the dosage administered and the patient's condition.

ADMINISTERED AS: powdered root, liquid extract.

Bittersweet *Solanum dulcamara.*

COMMON NAME: woody nightshade, violet bloom, scarlet berry, felonwood, felonwort, dulcamara.

OCCURRENCE: a climbing plant found in hedgerows in Britain.

PARTS USED: the twigs and root-bark. The twigs contain the alkaloid solamine and the glucoside dulcamarine which gives bittersweet its characteristic taste. It also contains sugar, gum, starch and resin.

MEDICINAL USES: narcotic, resolvent, diuretic and alterative. Bittersweet promotes all secretions, particularly of the skin and kidneys, and is generally used to clear up stubborn skin infections and eruptions, scrofula and ulcers and has been recommended in chronic bronchial catarrh, asthma or whooping cough. In large doses, the drug can cause paralysis of the central nervous system and lead to death.

ADMINISTERED AS: a fluid extract, decoction.

Blackberry *Rubus fructicosus.*

COMMON NAME: bramble, bumble-kite, bramble-kite, bly, brummel, brameberry, scaldhead, brambleberry.

OCCURRENCE: common throughout Britain in hedgerows and ditches.

PARTS USED: the root and leaves, which both contain tannin.
MEDICINAL USES: as astringent and tonic. It is valuable against dysentery and diarrhoea. A decoction of the root was used to treat whooping cough. A cordial or vinegar drink was made and is useful in treating looseness of the bowels, piles or a feverish cold.
ADMINISTERED AS: decoction, fluid extract or made into cordial, wine or vinegar.

Blackcurrant *Ribes nigrum.*
COMMON NAME: quinsy berries, squinancy berries.
OCCURRENCE: a common garden plant throughout Britain, but is only truly native to Yorkshire and the Lake District. It is also found in Europe.
PARTS USED: the fruit, leaves, bark and root.
MEDICINAL USES: diuretic, diaphoretic, febrifuge, refrigerant, detergent. The fruit juice is excellent in febrile diseases and can be made to an extract which is good for sore throats. The leaves when infused are cleansing while a root infusion is used in eruptive fevers and has been used to treat cattle. A decoction of the bark is effective against calculus, oedema and haemorrhoids. The fruit was commonly used to make jelly, wine and cheese.
ADMINISTERED AS: juice, infusion or decoction.

Black root *Leptandra virginica.*
COMMON NAME: culver's root, culver's physic, physic root, leptandra-wurzel, *Veronica virginica, Veronica purpurea, Paederota virginica, Eustachya purpurea, Eustachya alba.*
OCCURRENCE: found in the eastern United States.
PARTS USED: the rhizome which contains a crystalline principle and an impure resin, which together are called leptandrin and are said to be the active principles.

MEDICINAL USES: violent cathartic, emetic, tonic, antiseptic, diaphoretic. The action of the root on the body depends upon whether the root is dried or fresh. Fresh root is violently cathartic and emetic in action while the dried root has milder effects. It is used to excite the liver and promote the secretion of bile without harming the bowels and it is a good stomach tonic of benefit to diarrhoea, dysentery, cholera and torpid liver problems. The fresh root, however, may induce abortion and gives rise to bloody stools, but a decoction of the fresh root is used for intermittent fevers. The dried root has been used successfully in leprosy, dropsy, cancer, pulmonary tuberculosis and malaria.
ADMINISTERED AS: powdered root, decoction and fluid extract.

Bladderwrack *Fucus vesiculosus.*
COMMON NAME: bladder fucus, seawrack, kelp ware, black-tang, cutweed, seetang, blasentang, meeriche.
OCCURRENCE: common around the coasts of the North Atlantic Ocean including Britain.
PARTS USED: the root, stem and leaves, the thallus. The seaweed contains a volatile oil, cellulose, mucilage, mannite, soda and iodine along with the bromine compounds of sodium and potassium.
MEDICINAL USES: a deobstruent, antifat. It has been used to cause weight loss and reduce obesity by stimulation of the thyroid gland. The wine made from grapes and dried fucus has been of benefit in diseases of the hip, joints and bones in children. It may also be applied externally as a poultice to treat enlarged glands.
ADMINISTERED AS: a liquid extract, decoction, infusion, fluid extract, or charcoal derived from *Fucus vesiculosus.*

Bloodroot *Sanguinaria candensis.*
COMMON NAME: Indian paint, tetterwort, red pucoon, red root, paucon, coon root, snakebite, sweet slumber.

OCCURRENCE: a spring flower found in woods from Canada to Florida and west to Arkansas and Nebraska in the United States.
PARTS USED: the rhizome. It has the alkaloids sanguinarine, chelerythrine, protropine and B. homochelidonine as its active components. Protropine is one of the most widely used opium alkaloids.
MEDICINAL USES: emetic, cathartic, expectorant, emmenagogue. The plant is of great benefit in dyspepsia, asthma, bronchitis, croup and pulmonary consumption. It can be used in heart disease, heart weakness and palpitations, nervous irritation, torpid liver, scrofula, dysentery and to lower the pulse rate. Externally, it can be applied to cure ringworm, fungal growths, ulcers, eczema and cancerous growths. Care must be taken as toxic doses of *Sanguinaria* can be deleterious to the person.
ADMINISTERED AS: fluid extract, tincture, powdered root and solid extract.

Bluebell *Scilla nutans*, *Hyacinthus nonscriptus.*
COMMON NAME: calverkeys, culverkeys, auld man's bell, ring-o'-bells, jacinth, wood bells, *agraphis nutans.*
OCCURRENCE: abundant in western Europe, Great Britain and Italy.
PARTS USED: the bulb, dried and powdered.
MEDICINAL USES: diuretic, styptic. This medicine is little used today but it was considered a very powerful remedy for leucorrhoea. It may also have been used to cure snake bite. The fresh bulbs are poisonous, so the plant is always used when dried.
ADMINISTERED AS: powdered bulb.

Blue flag *Iris versicolor.*
COMMON NAME: poison flag, flag lily, liver lily, snake lily, dragon flower, dagger flower, water flag.
OCCURRENCE: indigenous to North America and was introduced into Britain and Europe and is now a common garden plant.

PARTS USED: the rhizome which contains starch, gum, tannin, isophthalic acid, salicylic acid and oleoresin of which the latter compound contains the medicinal properties.
MEDICINAL USES: alterative, diuretic, cathartic, stimulant. It is chiefly used for its alterative properties being useful as a purgative in disorders of the liver and the duodenum. Also, combined with other herbs as a blood purifier, or used alone against syphilis, scrofula, skin afflictions and dropsy.
ADMINISTERED AS: powdered root, solid extract, fluid extract or tincture.

Bogbean *Menyanthes trifoliata.*
COMMON NAME: buckbean, marsh trefoil, water trefoil, marsh clover, boonan.
OCCURRENCE: found in spongy bogs, marshes and shallow water throughout Europe and is more common in northern England and Scotland.
PARTS USED: the herb which consists of volatile oil and a glucoside called menyanthin.
MEDICINAL USES: as a tonic, cathartic, deobstruent and febrifuge. A liquid extract is used to treat rheumatism, scurvy and skin complaints. It has also been recommended as an external application to reduce glandular swelling. In the Highlands of Scotland it was used to remedy stomach pains, particularly due to ulcers, and bogbean was also brewed into beer and smoked as herb tobacco. It is thought to cure ague (malaria) where all other cures have failed.
ADMINISTERED AS: the liquid extract, infusion or as tea.

Boneset *Eupatonium perfoliatum.*
COMMON NAME: thoroughwort, Indian sage, feverwort.
OCCURRENCE: found in meadows and damp ground in North America and Europe.

PARTS USED: the herb. The important constituents are volatile oil, tannic acid, gum, resin, sugar and the glucoside eupatonin.
MEDICINAL USES: a diaphoretic, tonic, febrifuge, expectorant, stimulant, and laxative. It is used successfully to treat rheumatism, colds and influenza, catarrh and skin diseases. It acts slowly on the stomach, liver, bowel and uterus but it has a persistent beneficial effect. In large doses it has an emetic and purgative effect.
ADMINISTERED AS: powdered herb, fluid extract and solid extract.

Borage *Borago officinalis*.
COMMON NAME: burrage.
OCCURRENCE: naturalised in Britain and Europe and is found in gardens, rubbish heaps and near houses.
PARTS USED: the leaves and flowers consist of potassium, calcium and mineral acids along with nitrogen salts.
MEDICINAL USES: diuretic, demulcent, emollient, refrigerant. It is effective in treating fevers and pulmonary complaints as it activates the kidneys. It is applied externally as a poultice against inflammation and swelling and has been developed into a cream which treats itch and skin complaints, e.g. eczema and psoriasis. The flowers may be eaten raw, candied or made into a conserve to strengthen people weakened by prolonged illness.
ADMINISTERED AS: an infusion, poultice or lotion.

Box *Buxus sempervirens*.
COMMON NAME: dudgeon.
OCCURRENCE: native to Europe and western Africa but was introduced into Great Britain and the USA.
PARTS USED: the wood and leaves. The bark contains chlorophyll, wax, resin and tallow along with carbonate, sulphate and phos-

phate compounds. The leaves contain three alkaloids—buxine, parabuxine and parabuxonidine, as well as tannin.
MEDICINAL USES: the wood is diaphoretic, narcotic and sedative in full doses. It is generally prepared as a decoction for rheumatism and syphilis. The tincture was thought to be a bitter tonic, antiperiodic and cured leprosy. A volatile oil distilled from the wood has been used in epilepsy, piles and toothache. The leaves are sudorific, alterative and cathartic when powdered. The powder is poisonous so thus it makes an excellent purgative, vermifuge and is anthelmintic.
ADMINISTERED AS: powdered leaves, tincture, distilled oil, and decoction.

Brooklime *Veronica beccabunga.*
COMMON NAME: water pimpernel, becky leaves, cow cress, horse cress, housewell grass, limewort, brooklembe, limpwort, wall-ink, water-pumpy, well-ink.
OCCURRENCE: very common in all parts of Great Britain.
PARTS USED: the herb. This plant contains tannin, a bitter principle, a volatile oil and sulphur.
MEDICINAL USES: alterative, diuretic. It is used as an infusion as an antiscorbutic and to treat impurities of the blood.
ADMINISTERED AS: infusion or poultice.

Broom *Cytisus scoparius.*
COMMON NAME: broom tops, Irish tops, basam, bizzom, browne, brum, bream, green broom.
OCCURRENCE: indigenous to England and commonly found on heathland throughout Britain, Europe and northern Asia.
PARTS USED: the young herbaceous tops which contain sparteine and scoparin as the active components.
MEDICINAL USES: diuretic and cathartic. The broom tops may be

used as a decoction or infusion to aid dropsy while if the tops are pressed and treated broom juice is obtained. This fluid extract is generally used in combination with other diuretic compounds. An infusion of broom, AGRIMONY and DANDELION root is excellent in remedying bladder, kidney and liver trouble. *Cytisus* should be used carefully as the sparteine has a strong effect on the heart and, depending upon dose, can cause weakness of the heart similar to that caused by HEMLOCK (*Conium maculatum*). Death can occur in extreme cases if the respiratory organ's activity is impaired.
ADMINISTERED AS: fluid extract and infusion.

Bryony, Black *Tamus communis.*
COMMON NAME: blackeye root.
OCCURRENCE: native to Great Britain, common in woods and hedges.
PARTS USED: the root.
MEDICINAL USES: as a rubefacient and diuretic. The drug is seldom used internally now due to its poisonous nature, but was formerly used to treat asthmatic complaints. Externally the fresh root is scraped, pulped and applied as a plaster to areas affected by gout, rheumatism or paralysis. A root pulp poultice was used on bruises and black eyes to remove discolouration from the skin. Chilblains were treated using a tincture made from the roots.
ADMINISTERED AS: a plaster, poultice, tincture, rarely as expressed juice.

Bryony, White *Bryonia dioica, Bryonia alba.*
COMMON NAME: English mandrake, wild vine, wild hops, lady's seal, tetterbury, wild nep, tamus.
OCCURRENCE: a native of Europe, frequently found in England but rare in Scotland.
PARTS USED: the root.
MEDICINAL USES: irritative, hydragogue, cathartic. It was previously used as a purgative drug but these and other uses have been dis-

continued on account of its highly irritant nature. It is still used in small doses for coughs, influenza, bronchitis and pneumonia. It is useful in cardiac disorders caused by gout or rheumatism and in malarial and contagious diseases. Care should be taken when used, due to its poisonous nature.
ADMINISTERED AS: liquid extract.

Buchu *Barosma betulina.*
COMMON NAME: bucco, *Diosma betulina.*
OCCURRENCE: found at the Cape of Good Hope in South Africa.
PARTS USED: the leaves, which contain volatile oil, mucilage and diosphenol. They are collected from wild plants and this is strictly controlled by the government.
MEDICINAL USES: diuretic, diaphoretic, stimulant. The plant has a direct effect on the urinary organs, benefiting gravel, inflammation and catarrh of the bladder, cystitis, nephritis and urethritis. It has been classed as an official medicine in Great Britain since 1821.
ADMINISTERED AS: fluid extract, tincture and solid extract.

Bugle *Ajuga reptans.*
COMMON NAME: common bugle, carpenter's herb, middle confound, middle comfrey, sicklewort, herb carpenter, bugula.
OCCURRENCE: abundant throughout Great Britain in damp pastures and woods.
PARTS USED: the herb.
MEDICINAL USES: bitter, astringent and aromatic. As an infusion this herb is considered very good in arresting haemorrhages, easing irritation and coughs. It acts in a similar way to that of FOXGLOVE (*Digitalis purpurea*) in lowering the pulse rate and is said to be one of the mildest and best narcotics in existence. It is also considered good for the bad effects of excessive drinking.
ADMINISTERED AS: a decoction and infusion.

Burdock *Artium lappa.*
COMMON NAME: lappa, fox's clote, thorny burr, beggar's buttons, cockle buttons, love leaves, philanthropium, personata, happy major, clot-bur.
OCCURRENCE: freely found in ditches and hedgerows throughout England and Europe but rare in Scotland.
PARTS USED: the root, herb and seeds (fruits). They contain the chemicals inulin, mucilage, sugar and tannic acid along with a crystalline glucoside, lappin.
MEDICINAL USES: alterative, diuretic and diaphoretic. It is an excellent blood purifier and very effective in remedying all skin diseases. The root is most powerful and has antiscorbutic properties which make it very useful for boils, scurvy and rheumatism. Also used as a wash for ulcers and a poultice for tumours, gouty swellings and bruises. An infusion of the leaves aids the stomach and eases indigestion. The tincture obtained from the seeds is a relaxant, demulcent and a tonic for the skin.
ADMINISTERED AS: a fluid extract, infusion, tincture and solid extract.

Burnet, Greater *Sanguisorba officinalis.*
COMMON NAME: garden burnet, common burnet, salad burnet.
OCCURRENCE: found in moist meadows and shady areas almost all over Europe and in British gardens.
PARTS USED: the herb and root.
MEDICINAL USES: astringent and tonic. Decoction of the whole herb is useful in haemorrhages. Both the herb and root are taken internally to treat abnormal discharges such as diarrhoea, dysentery and leucorrhoea. It is also used to make herb beer.
ADMINISTERED AS: a powder and infusion.

Burr Marigold *Bidens Impartica.*
COMMON NAME: water agrimony.

OCCURRENCE: commonly found in wet places in England but less frequently seen in Scotland.
PARTS USED: the whole plant.
MEDICINAL USES: astringent, diaphoretic, diuretic. This plant has been useful in dropsy, gout, haematuria and fevers. It is very good in treating diseases of the respiratory organs where bleeding occurs and also in uterine haemorrhage.
ADMINISTERED AS: an infusion.

Butcher's Broom *Ruscus aculeatus.*
COMMON NAME: kneeholm, knee holy, jew's myrtle, sweet broom, pettigree.
OCCURRENCE: a low shrubby plant found in woods and waste ground, primarily in the south of England.
PARTS USED: the herb and root.
MEDICINAL USES: diaphoretic, diuretic, deobstruent and aperient. It is used in jaundice, gravel, urinary and female obstructions and is said to be good in clearing phlegm from the chest and relieving difficult breathing.
ADMINISTERED AS: a decoction.

Butterbur *Petasites vulgaris.*
COMMON NAME: langwort, umbrella plant, bog rhubarb, plapperdock, blatterdock, capdockin, bogshorns, butterdock.
OCCURRENCE: in low wet grounds, marshy meadows and riversides in Great Britain.
PARTS USED: the rhizome or rootstock.
MEDICINAL USES: as a cardiac tonic, a stimulant and diuretic. It is good as a remedy for fevers, asthma, colds, urinary complaints, gravel and plague. It is also taken as a homoeopathic remedy for severe neuralgia in the back and loins. Recently, the use of butterbur has been recommended in easing the pain of migraine and painful

menstruation. One of the most important developments is the treatment of cancer with *Petasites* when the drug attacks tumours and abnormal cell changes very strongly. In clinical tests, it has been shown to slow or stop the cancer spreading through the body. It has also become an effective remedy for severe asthma.
ADMINISTERED AS: a decoction and tincture.

Buttercup, Bulbous *Ranunculus bulbosus.*
COMMON NAME: St Antony's turnip, crowfoot, frogsfoot, goldcup.
OCCURRENCE: found in meadows and fields throughout Britain.
PARTS USED: the juice and herbs.
MEDICINAL USES: this plant has various uses including easing headaches and as a cure for shingles. The herb inflames and blisters the skin upon contact and is used to aid gout, sciatica and rheumatism. It has also been used as a poultice on the stomach.
ADMINISTERED AS: a poultice, decoction and tincture.

Cacao *Theobroma cacao.*
COMMON NAME: cocoa, chocolate tree.
OCCURRENCE: found in tropical America and cultivated in most tropical countries, e.g. Sri Lanka and Java.
PARTS USED: the seeds, which contain about two per cent of the chemical theobromine and forty to sixty per cent solid fat.
MEDICINAL USES: emollient, diuretic, stimulant and nutritive. The seeds are ground into a paste between hot rollers, with sugar and starch being added to produce cocoa. The cocoa butter (or oil of theobroma) produced forms a hard solid which is used in cosmetics, suppositories and coating pills. It has very good emollient qualities and is used to soften chapped hands and lips. The alkaloid, theobromine, which is contained in the beans is similar to caffeine in action on the central nervous system, but less power-

ful. It acts on the heart, kidneys and muscle and is used as a diuretic and stimulant of the kidneys. This is useful after fluid has accumulated in the body after heart failure and it is given in conjunction with digitalis (FOXGLOVE). The drug is also of benefit in high blood pressure.
ADMINISTERED AS: expressed oil, theobromine.

Calamint *Calamintha officinalis.*
COMMON NAME: mill mountain, mountain balm, basil thyme, mountain mint.
OCCURRENCE: a bushy plant found in hedgerows and lanes all over Great Britain and Europe.
PARTS USED: the herb. This contains a camphoraceous, volatile, stimulating oil similar to those found in other mint plants.
MEDICINAL USES: diaphoretic, expectorant and aromatic. It can be infused into a tea to treat weak stomachs, colic and flatulence. Can also be brewed into a syrup or decoction to heal the spleen, gall bladder and jaundice.
ADMINISTERED AS: an infusion, decoction and syrup.

Calamus *Aconus calamus.*
COMMON NAME: sweet flag, sweet sedge, sweet root, gladdon, sweet rush, sweet cane, myrtle grass, sweet myrtle, cinnamon sedge, myrtle wedge.
OCCURRENCE: grows freely in all European countries except Spain and it is common on river banks in Great Britain.
PARTS USED: the rhizome, which produces a volatile oil after steam distillation, which is made up of pinene and asaryl aldehyde. It also contains alkaloidal material including choline and the glucoside acorin.
MEDICINAL USES: aromatic, carminative, stimulant, tonic and stomachic. It is used to remove the discomfort of flatulence, wind,

colic, ague and dyspepsia. It can increase the appetite and aid digestion. Calamus oil is used in inhalations.
ADMINISTERED AS: a fluid extract, infusion, tincture and distilled oil.

Calotrophis *Calotrophis procera, Calotrophis gigantea.*
COMMON NAME: mudar bark, mudar yercum, *Asclepias onocera.*
OCCURRENCE: native to India but is cultivated in the East and West Indies and Sri Lanka.
PARTS USED: the dried bark. This contains several chemicals including madaralbum, madarfluavil, caoutchouc, mudarine, two resins and calatrophin which is an active poison similar to digitalis (FOXGLOVE).
MEDICINAL USES: in India, it is used as a remedy for elephantiasis, leprosy and chronic eczema. It may be taken internally for diarrhoea and dysentery. It has also been used to induce abortion and as a means of suicide. Atropine (from BELLADONNA, *Atropa belladonna*) may be used as an antidote to poisoning with calotrophis.
ADMINISTERED AS: powdered bark, tincture.

Calumba *jateorhiza calumba.*
COMMON NAME: *Cocculus palmatus*, colombo, *jateorhiza palmata.*
OCCURRENCE: indigenous to the forests of Mozambique and found throughout East Africa.
PARTS USED: the dried root. It contains three alkaloids—columbamine, jateorhizine and palmatine, which are closely related to berberine (from BARBERRY). There is also the crystalline principle, columbine, starch and mucilage in the root.
MEDICINAL USES: bitter tonic, febrifuge. Due to its lack of astringent qualities, it does not cause nausea, headache, sickness or fevers as other similar remedies do. It is very good against pulmonary consumption, weakness of the digestive organs, dysentery and for flatu-

lence in combination with GINGER and SENNA. Calumba can stop sickness in pregnancy and gastric irritation.
ADMINISTERED AS: cold infusion, tincture, fluid extract, powdered root, solid extract.

Camphor *Cinnamonum camphora.*
COMMON NAME: gum Camphor, laurel camphor, camphire, *Laurus camphora, Camphora officinarum.*
OCCURRENCE: found in China, Japan and parts of East Asia.
PARTS USED: the gum and distilled oil.
MEDICINAL USES: sedative, anodyne, antispasmodic, diaphoretic, anthelmintic, aromatic. It is mainly used in colds, chills, fevers, inflammatory complaints and for severe diarrhoea. It is taken internally for hysteria, nervousness, neuralgia and is used as an excitant in cases of heart failure due to infections, fevers and pneumonia. Camphor is highly valued in all irritations of the sexual organs. Large doses of camphor should be avoided as they can cause vomiting, palpitations and convulsions due to the effects it has on the human brain.
ADMINISTERED AS: tincture, distilled oil, injection, capsules.

Caraway *Carum Carvi.*
COMMON NAME: caraway seed, caraway fruit, alcaravea.
OCCURRENCE: common in Europe and Asia. Naturalized in Britain.
PARTS USED: the fruit, which produces a volatile oil containing a hydrocarbon, carvene and an oxygenated oil, carvol.
MEDICINAL USES: aromatic, stimulant and carminative. It was widely used as a cordial to ease dyspepsia and hysteria. The oil is applied to treat flatulence and stomach disorders. Distilled caraway water is used to ease flatulent colic in infants and is an excellent children's medicine. The bruised fruits were used to remove pain from bad earache and was also used as a poultice to take away

bruises. Caraway is widely used as a flavouring for cheeses and seed-cakes.
ADMINISTERED AS: a liquid extract and poultice.

Cardamom *Elettaria cardamomum.*
COMMON NAME: mysore cardamon seeds, malabar cardamom, ebil, kakelah seghar, capalaga, gujalatti elachi, ilachi, ailum, *Amomum cardamomum, A. repens, Alpina cardamom, matonia Cardamomum, Cardamomum minus, Cardamomi Semina.*
OCCURRENCE: native to southern India and cultivated in Sri Lanka.
PARTS USED: the dried ripe seed containing volatile and fixed oil, starch, mucilage, potassium salts, resin and lignin.
MEDICINAL USES: carminative, stimulant, aromatic. They have a warming aromatic effect which is useful in indigestion and flat-ulence. If chewed, they are said to be good for colic and head-aches. Cardamom is used chiefly as a flavouring for cakes, liqueurs, etc. and forms part of curry powder mixtures used in cookery.
ADMINISTERED AS: powdered seeds, tincture and fluid extract.

Caroba *Jacaranda procera.*
COMMON NAME: carob tree, carobinha, caaroba, *jacaranda caroba, Bignonia caroba.*
OCCURRENCE: found in South America and South Africa.
PARTS USED: the leaves contain many compounds including caroba balsam, caroborelinic acid, carobic acid, steocarobic acid, caroban and carobin.
MEDICINAL USES: alterative, diaphoretic, diuretic. The active principles have proved to be of benefit in treating syphilis and other venereal diseases. The soothing qualities of the herb have also been used to help epilepsy, as it has a sedative effect upon the nervous system. Caroba is rarely used in medicine today.
ADMINISTERED AS: dried, powdered leaves.

Carrot *Daucus carota.*
COMMON NAME: philtron, bird's nest, bee's nest.
OCCURRENCE: a native wild plant common everywhere in Great Britain. The wild and cultivated parts both exist today.
PARTS USED: the whole herb, seeds and root.
MEDICINAL USES: diuretic, stimulant, deobstruent. The herb infused in water is an active remedy in treating dropsy, chronic kidney infections and bladder disorders. Carrot tea was good for gout, while a strong decoction is good against gravel and flatulence. The roots have antiseptic properties and were formerly used as a laxative, vermifuge or a poultice. The wild carrot was particularly well thought of as a poultice for cancerous sores, while the seeds act in a similar manner to CARAWAY in treating stomach and gastric complaints. Carrot seed also has properties as an emmenagogue and in clearing obstructions of the viscera and jaundice. Carrots are made into jam, wine, spirit and can be roasted to produce a coffee substitute.
ADMINISTERED AS: an infusion, tea and poultice.

Cassia *Cinnamomum cassia.*
COMMON NAME: bastard cinnamon, Chinese cinnamon, cassia bark, canton cassia, *Cassia lignea*, *Cassia aromaticum.*
OCCURRENCE: indigenous to China and cultivated in Japan, Sumatra, Java, South America, Mexico and Sri Lanka.
PARTS USED: the bark. The bark of this tree is regarded as a substitute for cinnamon and it produces a volatile oil similar to oil of cinnamon. Cassia oil contains cinnamic aldehyde, cinnamylacetate, cinnamic acid, tannic acid and starch amongst other compounds.
MEDICINAL USES: stomachic, carminative, tonic, astringent and emmenagogue. The tincture is used in uterine haemorrhage, menorrhagia and to decrease the flow of breast milk. It is also

used to assist and flavour other drugs and benefits diarrhoea, vomiting, nausea and flatulence. Cassia oil is a powerful germicide but is not normally used in medicine as such as it is very irritant. It may be used for gastric pain, flatulent colic and gastric debility as it is a strong local stimulant.
ADMINISTERED AS: expressed oil, powdered bark.

Castor oil plant *Ricinus communis.*
COMMON NAME: palma Christi, castor oil bush.
OCCURRENCE: a native of India, but has been cultivated in many tropical, sub-tropical and temperate countries around the globe.
PARTS USED: the oil expressed from the seeds.
MEDICINAL USES: cathartic, purgative, laxative, vermifuge, galactogogue. Castor oil is regarded as one of the best laxative and purgative preparations available. It is of particular benefit for children and pregnant women due to its mild action in easing constipation, colic and diarrhoea due to slow digestion. The oil expels worms from the body, after other suitable remedies have been given. When applied externally, castor oil eases cutaneous complaints such as ringworm, itch and leprosy, while it is used as a carrier oil for solutions of pure alkaloids, e.g. atropine or cocaine, from BELLADONNA (*Atropa belladonna*), so that these drugs can be used in eye surgery. Castor oil is used for a range of industrial purposes from soap-making to varnishes.
ADMINISTERED AS: expressed oil.

Catmint *Nepeta cataria.*
COMMON NAME: catnep, nep.
OCCURRENCE: a wild English plant in hedges, field borders and waste ground. It is found on a localized basis in Scotland.
PARTS USED: the herb.

MEDICINAL USES: carminative, tonic, diaphoretic, refrigerant, mildly stimulating and slightly emmenagogue. This herb is good in treating colds, fevers, restlessness and colic. It is also used in nervousness and insanity and to calm children and soothe nightmares when taken as an infusion or conserve. Catmint can be applied to swellings and bruises as a poultice.
ADMINISTERED AS: an infusion, injection or poultice.

Cayenne *Capsicum minimum, Capsicum frutescens.*
COMMON NAME: African pepper, chillies, bird pepper.
OCCURRENCE: native to Zanzibar but is now cultivated in most tropical and sub-tropical countries, e.g. Sierra Leone, Japan and Madagascar.
PARTS USED: the fruit, both fresh and dried.
MEDICINAL USES: stimulant, tonic, carminative, rubefacient. It is possibly the purest and best stimulant in herbal medicine. It produces natural warmth and helps the blood circulation, and eases weakness of the stomach and intestines. Cayenne is added to tonics and is said to ward off disease and can prevent development of colds and fevers.
ADMINISTERED AS: powdered fruit, tincture, capsules, dietary item.

Cedar, Yellow *Thuja occidentalis.*
COMMON NAME: tree of life, arbor vitae, false white cedar, *Cedrus lycea*, hackmatack, thuia de Canada, Lebensbaum.
OCCURRENCE: the United States and Canada.
PARTS USED: the leaves and twigs. The plant contains the bitter principle pinipicrin, volatile oil, sugar, wax, resin and a colouring principle called thujin. The leaves and twigs yield an essential oil similar to camphor, which contains pinene, fenchone, thujone and carvone.
MEDICINAL USES: aromatic, astringent, diuretic, anthelmintic, irri-

tant, expectorant, emmenagogue. A decoction of the twigs can help intermittent fevers, coughs, gout, amenorrhoea, dropsy and scurvy. When made into an ointment, the leaves ease rheumatism. An infusion is good at removing warts and fungal growths. A preparation of the twigs may induce abortion by reflex action on the uterus from severe gastro-intestinal irritation. This plant should be used with some care.
ADMINISTERED AS: infusion, decoction, injection, poultice, tincture, ointment.

Celandine *Chelidonium majus.*
COMMON NAME: garden celandine, common celandine, greater celandine.
OCCURRENCE: common all over Great Britain and Europe.
PARTS USED: the herb, which contains the alkaloids chelidanine, chelerythrin (of which the latter is narcotic), homochelidonine A and B. Three other major chemicals are found in the plant.
MEDICINAL USES: alterative, diuretic and purgative. It is of benefit to jaundice, eczema, scrofulous diseases and scurvy. The fresh juice was used to cure warts, ringworm and corns but should not otherwise be allowed to come into direct contact with the skin. In various forms, it has previously been effective against itching, piles, toothache and cancer.
ADMINISTERED AS: infusion, fluid extract, decoction, lotion, poultice.

Celery *Apium graveolens.*
COMMON NAME: smallage, wild celery.
OCCURRENCE: native to southern Europe and cultivated in Britain.
PARTS USED: the ripe seeds, herb and root of which the seeds contain two oils and apiol.
MEDICINAL USES: carminative, stimulant, diuretic, tonic, nervine and aphrodisiac. It is utilised as a tonic in combination with other herbs,

promoting restfulness, sleep and lack of hysteria and is excellent in relieving rheumatism.
ADMINISTERED AS: fluid extract, essential oil and powdered seeds.

Chamomile *Anthemis nobilis.*
COMMON NAME: Roman chamomile, double chamomile, manzanilla (Spanish), maythen (Saxon).
OCCURRENCE: a low growing plant found wild in the British Isles.
PARTS USED: the flowers and herb. The active principles therein are a volatile oil, anthemic acid, tannic acid and a glucoside.
MEDICINAL USES: tonic, stomachic, anodyne and anti-spasmodic. An infusion of chamomile tea is an extremely effective remedy for hysterical and nervous afflictions in women, as well as an emmenagogue. Chamomile has a powerful soothing and sedative effect which is harmless. A tincture is used to cure diarrhoea in children and it is used with purgatives to prevent griping, and as a tonic it helps dropsy. Externally, it can be applied alone or with other herbs as a poultice to relieve pain, swellings, inflammation and neuralgia. Its strong antiseptic properties make it invaluable for reducing swelling of the face due to abscess or injury. As a lotion, the flowers are good for resolving toothache and earache. The herb itself is an ingredient in herb beers. The use of chamomile can be dated back to ancient Egyptian times when they dedicated the plant to the sun because of its extensive healing properties.
ADMINISTERED AS: decoction, infusion, fluid extract and essential oil.

Cherry laurel *Prunus laurocerasus.*
OCCURRENCE: native to Russia and now cultivated in many temperate European countries.
PARTS USED: the leaves. The main constituent is prulaurasin which resembles amygdalin and hydrocyanic acid.

MEDICINAL USES: sedative, narcotic. The leaves are used to produce a distilled water which is the main herbal preparation used of this herb. It is good against coughs, dyspepsia, indigestion, whooping cough and asthma.
ADMINISTERED AS: cherry laurel water.

Chestnut, Horse *Aesculus hippocastanum.*
COMMON NAME: *Hippocastanum vulgare.*
OCCURRENCE: a tree native to northern and central Asia from which it was introduced into England and Scotland.
PARTS USED: the bark and fruit, from both of which a fluid extract is made.
MEDICINAL USES: tonic, narcotic, febrifuge and astringent. The bark is used in intermittent fevers as an infusion. It is also used externally to treat ulcers. The fruits are employed in easing neuralgia, rheumatism as well as rectal complaints and haemorrhoids.
ADMINISTERED AS: an infusion and fluid extract.

Chestnut, Sweet *Castanea vesca.*
COMMON NAME: *Fagus castanea*, sardia nut, Jupiter's nut, hushed nut, Spanish chestnut, *Castanea vulgaris.*
OCCURRENCE: very common in Britain, Europe and North America.
PARTS USED: the leaves.
MEDICINAL USES: tonic, astringent. It is used in a popular remedy to treat fever and ague. Its reputation is due to the great effectiveness in treating violent and convulsive coughs, particularly whooping cough and in other irritable respiratory organ conditions. The nut is commonly eaten as food or as a stuffing for meat.
ADMINISTERED AS: an infusion.

Chickweed *Stellania media.*
COMMON NAME: starweed, star chickweed, *Alsine media*, passerina.

OCCURRENCE: native to all temperate and North Arctic regions and is naturalized wherever Man has settled. A common weed.
PARTS USED: the whole herb, both fresh and dried.
MEDICINAL USES: demulcent, refrigerant. It is good as a poultice to reduce inflammation and heal indolent ulcers, but is most important as an ointment in treating eye problems and cutaneous diseases. It will also benefit scurvy and kidney disorders as an infusion.
ADMINISTERED AS: an infusion, poultice and ointment.

Chicory *Cichonium intybus.*
COMMON NAME: succory, wild succory, hendibeh, barbe de capucin.
OCCURRENCE: common in England and Ireland but rarer in Scotland.
PARTS USED: the root.
MEDICINAL USES: tonic, diuretic and laxative. A decoction of the root has benefit in jaundice, liver problems, gout and rheumatic complaints. The root, when dried, roasted and ground, may be added to coffee or may be drunk on its own as a beverage.
ADMINISTERED AS: a decoction, poultice, syrup or distilled water.

Chives *Allium schoenoprasum.*
COMMON NAME: cives.
OCCURRENCE: native to temperate and northern Europe and Great Britain. Cultivated over a large area of the northern hemisphere.
PARTS USED: the herb.
MEDICINAL USES: this herb stimulates the appetite and helps digestion during convalescence. It is also said to be effective against infections and to prevent anaemia. They are also widely used in food dishes and add vitamins and colour to many meals.
ADMINISTERED AS: fresh herbs.

Cicely, Sweet *Myrrhis odorata.*
COMMON NAME: smooth cicely, British myrrh, anise, great sweet cher-

vil, smelt chervil, sweet bracken, sweet-fern, sweet humlock, sweets, the Roman plant, shepherd's needle, cow chervil.
OCCURRENCE: native to Great Britain and also found in mountain pastures across Europe.
PARTS USED: the root and herb.
MEDICINAL USES: aromatic, carminative, stomachic, expectorant. The fresh root may be eaten or used as a tonic in brandy. It eases coughs, flatulence, indigestion and stomach upsets. The herb, as an infusion, is good for anaemia and a tonic for young girls. The antiseptic roots have been used for snake or dog bites while the distilled water is diuretic and effective in treating pleurisy. Sweet cicely essence is said to have aphrodisiac properties.
ADMINISTERED AS: a root infusion, herb infusion, decoction, essence and distilled water.

Cinnamon *Cinnamomum zeylanicum.*
COMMON NAME: *Lauris cinnamomum.*
OCCURRENCE: native to Sri Lanka but is cultivated in other Eastern countries.
PARTS USED: the bark.
MEDICINAL USES: carminative, astringent, stimulant, antiseptic, aromatic. It is used as a local stimulant as a powder and infusion, generally combined with other herbs. Cinnamon stops vomiting and nausea, relieves flatulence and diarrhoea and can also be employed to stop haemorrhage of the womb.
ADMINISTERED AS: powder, distilled water, tincture or essential oil.

Clematis *Clematis recta.*
COMMON NAME: upright virgin's bower, *Clammula jovis.*
OCCURRENCE: a perennial plant common to Europe.
PARTS USED: the roots and stem.
MEDICINAL USES: diuretic, diaphoretic. When bruised, the leaves

and flowers irritate the eyes and throat prompting tears and coughing. If applied to the skin, it produces inflammation and blisters appear. The herb is used both as a local external application, and internally against syphilis, cancer and other ulcers. It is used by homoeopaths for eye complaints, gonorrhoea and inflammatory conditions.
ADMINISTERED AS: dried leaves, fluid extract.

Clivers *Galium aparine.*
COMMON NAME: cleavers, goosegrass, borweed, hedgesheriff, hayriffe, eriffe, grip grass, hayruff, catchweed, scratweed, mutton chops, robin-run-in-the-grass, love-man, goosebill, everlasting friendship.
OCCURRENCE: an abundant hedgerow weed in Europe, Great Britain and North America.
PARTS USED: the herb, which contains chlorophyll, starch, galitannic acid, citric acid and rubichloric acid.
MEDICINAL USES: diuretic, tonic, aperient and alterative. It is successfully administered to treat obstruction of the urinary organs, gravel, suppression of urine, etc. A wash of the herb helps sunburn and freckles, while an ointment provides benefit against cancerous growths and tumours. The expressed juice or infusion will help scurvy, scrofula, psoriasis and other skin complaints as well as stopping insomnia and inducing sleep.
ADMINISTERED AS: an infusion, decoction, ointment, expressed juice or lotion.

Clover, Red *Trifolium pratense.*
COMMON NAME: trefoil, purple clover.
OCCURRENCE: widely distributed in Britain and Europe.
PARTS USED: the flowers.
MEDICINAL USES: alterative, sedative, antispasmodic. The fluid ex-

tract or infusion are excellent in treating bronchial and whooping coughs. External applications of the herb in a poultice have been used on cancerous growths.
ADMINISTERED AS: fluid extract and infusion.

Clove *Eugenia caryophyllata.*
COMMON NAME: *Eugenia aromatica*, *Eugenia caryophyllus*, clavos.
OCCURRENCE: grows on the Molucca Islands in the southern Philippines.
PARTS USED: the underdeveloped flowers.
MEDICINAL USES: stimulating, carminative, aromatic. It is given as powder or an infusion for nausea, vomiting, flatulence, languid indigestion and dyspepsia. The volatile oil contains the medicinal properties and it is a strong germicide, antiseptic and a local irritant. It has been used as an expectorant to aid bronchial troubles. Clove oil is often used in association with other medicines.
ADMINISTERED AS: powdered cloves, infusion, essential oil, fluid extract.

Club moss *Lycopodium clavatum.*
COMMON NAME: lycopodium, lycopodium seed, vegetable sulphur, wolf's claw, muscus terrestris repens.
OCCURRENCE: occurs throughout Great Britain being most plentiful on heath or moorland in northern countries and is also found all over the world.
PARTS USED: the fresh plant and spores.
MEDICINAL USES: spores are diuretic, nervine and aperient. The fresh plant has been used as a stomachic and a diuretic herb in calculus and kidney complaints. The spores are currently applied externally to wounds and taken internally for diarrhoea, dysentery, gout and scurvy.
ADMINISTERED AS: dried spores, fresh moss.

Coca, Bolivian: *Erythroxylum coca*; **Peruvian**: *Erythroxylum truxillense*.

COMMON NAME: cuca, cocaine.

OCCURRENCE: native to Peru and Bolivia; cultivated in Java and Sri Lanka.

PARTS USED: the leaves. They contain the alkaloids cocaine, amamyl cocaine and truxilline or cocamine when grown in South America. Eastern-grown plants contain additional chemicals and glucosides.

MEDICINAL USES: nerve stimulant, anodyne, tonic, aphrodisiac. The leaves are used as a cerebral and muscle stimulant during convalescence relieving nausea, vomiting and stomach pains. It is utilized as a general nerve tonic and in treating asthma. In South America, the locals chew the leaves to relieve hunger and fatigue, but this does cause health damage when done over a long period of time. There is a danger of developing an addictive habit to this drug and the possible medicinal benefits are less than the potential health damage. People with a cocaine habit can appear emaciated, suffer loss of memory, sleeplessness and delusions. In Great Britain, the distribution and use of this drug is controlled by the Dangerous Drugs Act.

ADMINISTERED AS: tincture, powdered leaves, fluid extract.

Coffee *Coffea arabica*.

COMMON NAME: caffea.

OCCURRENCE: native to a province of Abyssinia and cultivated throughout the tropics.

PARTS USED: the seed and leaves. When roasted, coffee contains oil, wax, caffeine, aromatic oil, tannic acid, caffetannic acid, gum, sugar and protein.

MEDICINAL USES: stimulant, diuretic, anti-narcotic, anti-emetic. Coffee is commonly used as a beverage but it can also be applied as a

medicine. It is a brain stimulant, causing sleeplessness and hence is useful in cases of narcotic poisoning. For this reason it is very good against snake bite in that it helps stop people falling into a coma. Caffeine can be valuable for heart disease and fluid retention and it is used against drunkenness. As a powerful diuretic, it can help ease gout, rheumatism, gravel and dropsy.
ADMINISTERED AS: beverage, caffeine preparation.

Cohosh, Black *Cimicifuga racemosa.*
COMMON NAME: black snakeroot, bugbane, rattleroot, rattleweed, squawroot, *Actaea racemosa*, *Macrotys actaeoides.*
OCCURRENCE: a native of the United States and Canada and was introduced into England around 1860.
PARTS USED: the rhizome. The main constituents are a resinous substance known as cimicifuga (or macrotin) and racemosin which gives the drug its bitter taste.
MEDICINAL USES: astringent, emmenagogue, diuretic, alterative, expectorant. This root is said to be effective in many disorders including whooping cough and rheumatism. It is supposed to be an antidote to poison and rattlesnake bites. The drug can help ease children's diarrhoea, and in consumption acts by slowing the pulse rate, inducing perspiration and easing the cough. In overdoses, black Cohosh can cause vomiting and nausea.
ADMINISTERED AS: tincture, infusion, decoction, powdered root.

Cohosh, Blue *Caulophyllum thalictroides.*
COMMON NAME: papoose root, squawroot, blueberry root, *Leontice thalichoides.*
OCCURRENCE: found in the United States and Canada.
PARTS USED: the rhizome. It contains gum, starch, salts, soluble resin and a chemical similar to saponin.
MEDICINAL USES: diuretic, antispasmodic, vermifuge, emmenagogue,

athelmintic, diaphoretic. This drug has been used in rheumatism, epilepsy, uterine inflammation, hysteria and dropsy. It is also taken to expedite childbirth and induce menstruation.
ADMINISTERED AS: decoction, infusion, tincture, solid extract.

Coltsfoot *Tussilago farfara.*
COMMON NAME: coughwort, hallfoot, horsehoof, ass's foot, foalswort, fieldhove, bullsfoot, donnhove.
OCCURRENCE: commonly found wild on waste ground and riverbanks in Great Britain.
PARTS USED: the leaves, flowers and root.
MEDICINAL USES: demulcent, expectorant and tonic. Coltsfoot is one of the most popular cough remedies and is generally taken in conjunction with HOREHOUND, MARSHMALLOW or GROUND IVY. It has been called "nature's best herb for the lungs" and it was recommended that the leaves be smoked to relieve a cough. Today, it forms the basis of British herb tobacco along with BOGBEAN, EYEBRIGHT, WOOD BETONY, ROSEMARY, THYME, LAVENDER and CHAMOMILE which is said to relieve asthma, catarrh, bronchitis and lung troubles.
ADMINISTERED AS: syrup or smoked when dried.

Columbine *Aquilegia vulgaris.*
COMMON NAME: culverwort.
OCCURRENCE: found as both a wild and garden plant in Great Britain.

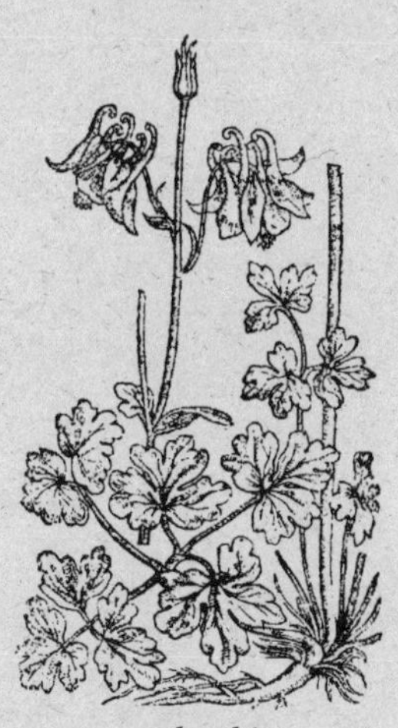

columbine

PARTS USED: the leaves, roots and seeds.
MEDICINAL USES: astringent. It must be administered in small doses where it is used as a lotion for sore mouths and throats. It was also used for stone, jaundice and liver obstructions. Large doses can cause poisoning, so care must be taken in utilizing this drug.
ADMINISTERED AS: fresh root and infusion.

Comfrey *Symphytum officinale*.
COMMON NAME: common comfrey, knitbone, knitback, bruisewort, slippery root, gum plant, consolida, ass ear, blackwort.
OCCURRENCE: a native of Europe and temperate Asia but common by rivers and ditches throughout England.
PARTS USED: the root and leaves. The roots contain a large quantity of mucilage, choline and allantoin.
MEDICINAL USES: demulcent, mildly astringent, expectorant and vulnerary. It is frequently used in pulmonary complaints, to soothe intestinal trouble and is a gentle remedy for diarrhoea and dysentery. A strong decoction or tea is administered in cases of internal haemorrhage whether it is the lungs, stomach, bowels or haemorrhoids. Externally, the leaves have been used as a poultice to promote healing of severe cuts, ulcers and abscesses and to reduce swelling, sprains and bruises. Allantoin is known to reduce swelling round damaged or fractured bones, thus allowing healing to occur faster and more thoroughly.
ADMINISTERED AS: a decoction, poultice and liquid extract.

Coolwort *Tiarella cordifolia*.
COMMON NAME: foam flower, mitrewort.
OCCURRENCE: found in North America from Canada to Virginia.
PARTS USED: the herb.
MEDICINAL USES: diuretic, tonic. Very good in cases of gravel, suppression of urine and other bladder diseases. It is taken as a tonic

in indigestion and dyspepsia where it corrects acidity and aids liver function.
ADMINISTERED AS: infusion, decoction.

Coriander *Coriandrum sativum.*
OCCURRENCE: indigenous to southern Europe and found occasionally in Britain, at riversides, fields and waste ground.
PARTS USED: the fruit and leaves.
MEDICINAL USES: stimulant, aromatic and carminative. It is generally used with active purgatives as flavouring and to lessen their griping tendencies. Coriander water was formerly used for windy colic.
ADMINISTERED AS: powdered fruit, fluid extract.

Corkwood tree *Duboisia myoporoides.*
COMMON NAME: duboisia.
OCCURRENCE: found in Australia in the states of New South Wales and Queensland.
PARTS USED: the leaves which contain alkaloidal sulphates, mainly hyoscyamine and hyoscine.
MEDICINAL USES: sedative, hypnotic, mydriatic. The drug aids the activity of the respiratory system and it is sometimes used as a replacement for atropine, from BELLADONNA (*Atropa belladonna*). The tincture of the drug is used in treating eye afflictions and paralysis.
ADMINISTERED AS: tincture.

Cornflower *Centaurea cyanus.*
COMMON NAME: bluebottle, bluebow, hurtsickle, blue cap, bluet.
OCCURRENCE: common in cultivated fields and roadsides in Britain.
PARTS USED: the flowers.
MEDICINAL USES: tonic, stimulant and emmenagogue properties. A

water distilled from cornflower petals was said to be a remedy for eye inflammation and weak eyesight.
ADMINISTERED AS: distilled water and infusion.

Costmary *Tanacetum balsamita.*
COMMON NAME: alecost, balsam herb, costmarie, mace, balsamita.
OCCURRENCE: an old English herb, naturalized from the Orient in the sixteenth century.
PARTS USED: the leaves.
MEDICINAL USES: formerly used as an aperient, antiseptic and astringent herb in treating dysentery. Used as an infusion to heal stomach and head problems. Also flavouring for ale and in salads.
ADMINISTERED AS: infusion and tincture.

Cotton root *Gossypium herbaceum* (and other species).
OCCURRENCE: indigenous to India and cultivated in Greece, Turkey, Sicily and Malta.
PARTS USED: the root-bark which contains a peculiar acid resin, sugar, gum, chlorophyll, fixed oil and tannin.
MEDICINAL USES: this drug is used to induce abortion or miscarriage as it causes contraction of the uterus. It is useful in treating abnormal uterine bleeding particularly when linked to fibroids, and in cases of difficult or obstructed menstruation. A preparation is given to induce labour (at full term) to aid safe delivery. It is said to be of use in sexual lassitude.
ADMINISTERED AS: fluid extract, decoction, solid extract.

Couchgrass *Agropyrum repens.*
COMMON NAME: twitchgrass, Scotch quelch, quickgrass, dog's grass, *Triticum repens.*
OCCURRENCE: abundant in fields and waste ground in Britain, Europe, northern Asia and North and South America.

PARTS USED: the rhizome, which contains triticin (a carbohydrate).
MEDICINAL USES: diuretic, demulcent, aperient. Widely used in complaints of the urinary organs and bladder. Also recommended for gout and rheumatism.
ADMINISTERED AS: an infusion, decoction and liquid extract.

Cowslip *Primula veris.*
COMMON NAME: herb Peter, paigle, peggle, key flower, key of heaven, fairy cups, petty mulleins, patsywort, plumrocks, mayflower, Our Lady's keys, arthritica.
OCCURRENCE: a common wild flower in all parts of Great Britain.
PARTS USED: the flower.
MEDICINAL USES: sedative, antispasmodic. It is very good in relieving restlessness and insomnia. Commonly brewed into a wine which was a good children's medicine in small doses.
ADMINISTERED AS: an infusion or wine.

Cramp bark *Viburnum opulus.*
COMMON NAME: guelder rose, snowball tree, king's crown, high cranberry, red elder, rose elder, may rose, whitsun rose, dog rowan tree, silver bells, whitsun bosses, gaitre berries, black haw.
OCCURRENCE: indigenous to Great Britain and North America, although rare in Scotland.
PARTS USED: the bark whose chief constituents are the glucoside viburnine, tannin, resin and valerianic acid.
MEDICINAL USES: antispasmodic, nervine, sedative. This drug is of benefit in all nervous complaints, debility, cramps and spasms of all types, asthma and hysteria. It has been effective in treating convulsions, fits, lockjaw, heart disease, palpitations and rheumatism.
ADMINISTERED AS: tincture, decoction, infusion, fluid extract.

Croton *Croton tiglian.*
Common name: tiglium, *Tiglium officinale*.
Occurrence: a tree found on the Malabar coast of India and on the Indian archipelago.
Parts used: the oil expressed from the seeds, croton oil contains glycerides of stearic, palmitic, myristic, lauric and oleic acids; the glycerin ethers of formic, acetic, isobutyric and isovaleranic acids. The active principle is probably Crotonic acid.
Medicinal uses: irritant, rubefacient, cathartic, purgative. A drastic purgative drug which acts quickly, often evacuating the bowels in less than one hour. In large doses, it causes vomiting and severe griping pains which can possibly be fatal. The drug is only used in cases of obstinate constipation where other drugs have failed. It is applied externally as a counter-irritant to relieve rheumatism, gout, neuralgia and bronchitis. The use of this oil should be monitored most carefully, only administered in small doses, and never given to children or pregnant women.
Administered as: expressed oil.

Crowfoot, Upright meadow *Ranunculus acris.*
Common name: gold cup, grenouillette.
Occurrence: native in meadows, pastures and fields in all parts of northern Europe and Great Britain.
Parts used: the whole herb.
Medicinal uses: the expressed juice is used to remove warts. A poultice of the fresh herb is good at removing violent, painful headaches or in relieving gout. The fresh herb once formed part of a famous cure for cancer practised in 1794.
Administered as: fresh leaves, expressed juice.

Cuckoopint *Arum maculatum.*
COMMON NAME: lords-and-ladies, starchwort, arum, adder's root, friar's cowl, kings and queens, parson and clerk, ramp, Quaker, wake robin.
OCCURRENCE: the sole British species of the arum, aroidae family and is also widely distributed over Europe.
PARTS USED: the root. This contains starch, albumen, sugar, lignin, saponin and an unidentified alkaloid.
MEDICINAL USES: diaphoretic, expectorant, diuretic, stimulant. The fresh root can be prepared into a tincture and given to remedy sore, feverish throats. The dried root can be stored for long periods, but is rarely employed as a medicine today. An ointment prepared of the fresh root was used to cure ringworm.
ADMINISTERED AS: tincture, expressed juice and ointment.

Cucumber *Cucumis sativa.*
COMMON NAME: cowcumber.
OCCURRENCE: a native of the East Indies, but was first cultivated in Britain around 1573.
PARTS USED: the whole fruit, peeled or unpeeled, raw and cooked.
MEDICINAL USES: the seeds are diuretic and are an excellent taeniacide and purge. The fruit is very good as a skin cosmetic as it has cooling, healing and soothing effects on irritated skin. Cucumber juice is widely utilised in emollient ointments or creams and is good for sunburn.
ADMINISTERED AS: expressed juice, lotion or ointment.

Cudweed *Graphalium uliginosum.*
COMMON NAME: cottonweed, marsh everlasting, cotton dawes.
OCCURRENCE: found in marshy areas in all parts of Europe.
PARTS USED: the herb.

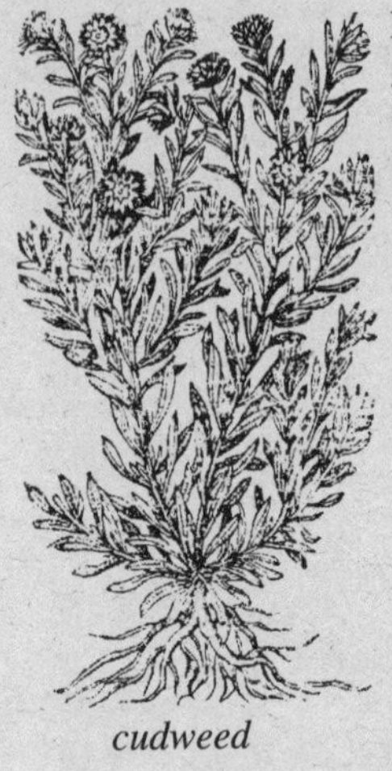
cudweed

MEDICINAL USES: astringent. It is a very good remedy for quinsy when used as a gargle and can also be taken internally.
ADMINISTERED AS: an infusion.

Cumin *Cuminum cyminum.*
COMMON NAME: cummin, *Cumino aigro.*
OCCURRENCE indigenous to upper Egypt and is cultivated in Arabia, India, China and Mediterranean countries since early times.
PARTS USED: the fruit. The chief constituents are a volatile oil, a fatty oil with resin, mucilage, gum, malates and albuminous matter.
MEDICINAL USES: stimulant, carminative, antispasmodic. This herb has similar effects to FENNEL and CARAWAY but its use has declined because of its disagreeable taste. It had a considerable reputation in helping correct flatulence caused by languid digestion and as a remedy for colic and dyspeptic headache. Applied externally as a plaster, it eased stitches and pains in the side and has been combined with other herbs to form a stimulating liniment.
ADMINISTERED AS: dried, powdered fruit, whole fruit.

Cup moss *Cladonia pyxidata.*
COMMON NAME: chin cups.
OCCURRENCE: indigenous to north-west America but is also a common weed through Great Britain and Europe.
PARTS USED: the whole plant.

MEDICINAL USES: expectorant—used as a decoction to treat children's coughs and whooping cough with great effectiveness.
ADMINISTERED AS: decoction.

Daffodil *Narcissus pseudo-narcissus.*
COMMON NAME: narcissus, porillion, daffy-down-dilly, fleur de coucou, Lent lily.
OCCURRENCE: found wild in most European countries including the British Isles.
PARTS USED: the bulb, leaves and flowers. The bulbs contain an alkaloid called lyconine.
MEDICINAL USES: the flowers, when powdered, have emetic properties and as an infusion are used in pulmonary catarrh. The bulbs are also emetic and, indeed, can cause people to collapse and die as a result of paralysis of the central nervous system caused by the action of lyconine, which acts quickly. Accidents have resulted from daffodil bulbs being mistaken for ONIONS and eaten. Since high temperatures and cooking does not break down the poisonous alkaloid, considerable care should be taken to avoid problems. The bulbs are used externally as an astringent poultice to dissolve hard swellings and aid wound healing.
ADMINISTERED AS: powder and extract.

Daisy, Ox-eye *Chrysanthemum leuconthemum.*
COMMON NAME: great ox-eye, goldens, marguerite, moon daisy, horse gowan, maudlin daisy, field daisy, dun daisy, butter daisy, horse daisy, maudlinwort, white weed, gowan.
OCCURRENCE: found in fields throughout Europe and northern Asia.
PARTS USED: the whole herb, flowers and root.
MEDICINAL USES: antispasmodic, diuretic, tonic. This herb's main use has been in whooping cough, asthma and nervous excitabil-

ity. When taken as a tonic, it acts in a similar way to CHAMOMILE flowers and calms night sweats and nightmares. An infusion of ox-eye daisy flowers is good at relieving bronchial coughs and catarrh. It is also used as a lotion for wounds, bruises and ulcers.
ADMINISTERED AS: an infusion and lotion.

Damiana *Turnera aphrodisiaca* or *Turnera diffusa* var. *aphrodisiaca.*
OCCURRENCE: indigenous to Texas and Mexico; cultivated in other areas of sub-tropical America and Africa.
PARTS USED: the leaves which contain a volatile oil, resins, tannin and the bitter principle damianin.
MEDICINAL USES: mild purgative, diuretic, tonic, stimulant, aphrodisiac. This drug acts as a tonic to the nervous system and has a direct and general beneficial effect on the reproductive organs.
ADMINISTERED AS: fluid extract, solid extract.

Dandelion *Taraxacum officinale.*
COMMON NAME: priest's crown, swine's snout.
OCCURRENCE: widely found across the northern temperate zone in pastures, meadows and waste ground.
PARTS USED: the root and leaves. The main constituents of the root are taraxacin, a bitter substance, and taraxacerin, an acid resin, along with the sugar inulin.
MEDICINAL USES: diuretic, tonic and slightly aperient. It acts as a general body stimulant but chiefly acts on the liver and kidneys. Dandelion is used as a bitter tonic in atonic dyspepsia as a mild laxative and to promote increased appetite and digestion. The herb is best used in combination with other herbs and is used in many patent medicines. Roasted dandelion root is also used as a coffee substitute and helps ease dyspepsia, gout and rheumatism.

ADMINISTERED AS: fluid and solid extract, decoction, infusion and tincture.

Dill *Peucedanum graveolus, Fructus anethi.*
COMMON NAME: dill seed, dill fruit, *Anethum graveolus, Fructus anethi.*
OCCURRENCE: indigenous to Mediterranean districts and South Russia and is cultivated in England and Europe.
PARTS USED: the dried ripe fruit. An oil obtained from the fruit is almost identical to oil of CARAWAY, both containing limonene and carvone.
MEDICINAL USES: stimulant, aromatic, carminative and stomachic. It is usually given as dillwater which is very good for children's flatulence or disordered digestion. Oil of dill is used in medicine in largely the same way, but is also used in perfuming soaps.
ADMINISTERED AS: distilled water, essential oil.

Dock, Yellow *Rumex crispus.*
COMMON NAME: curled dock.
OCCURRENCE: normally found on roadside ditches and waste ground, all over Great Britain.
PARTS USED: the root and whole herb.
MEDICINAL USES: the root has laxative, alterative and a mildly tonic action and is used in rheumatism, bilious complaints and haemorrhoids. It is very useful in treating jaundice, diseases of the blood, scurvy, chronic skin diseases and as a tonic on the digestive system. Yellow dock is said to have a positive effect on slowing the development of cancer, because of its alterative and tonic properties. It has similar effects to that of RHUBARB and has been used in treating diphtheria.
ADMINISTERED AS: dried extract, syrup, infusion, tincture, ointment, fluid extract and solid extract.

Dodder *Cuscuta europea.*
COMMON NAME: lesser dodder, dodder of thyme, beggarweed, hellweed, strangle tare, scaldweed, devil's guts.
OCCURRENCE: a parasitic plant found in most areas of the world.
PARTS USED: the herb.
MEDICINAL USES: hepatic, laxative, purgative. A decoction made with dodder, GINGER and ALLSPICE has been used against urinary complaints, kidney, spleen and liver disorders. The herb is good in treating sciatica, scorbutic problems, scrofulous tumours and it acts as a purge due to its very bitter taste.
ADMINISTERED AS: decoction, infusion.

Dog-rose *Rosa canina.*
COMMON NAME: wild briar, hip tree, cynosbatos.
OCCURRENCE: indigenous to Great Britain.
PARTS USED: the ripe fruit which contain invert fruit sugars, a range of mineral salts and a large proportion of vitamin C or ascorbic acid.
MEDICINAL USES: astringent, refrigerant and pectoral. The fruit is used in strengthening the stomach and digestion, as well as easing coughs. It is made into an uncooked preserve, a syrup which is excellent for infants and children and rose-hip tea has very beneficial effects. An infusion of dog-rose leaves has been used as a tea substitute and has a pleasant aroma.
ADMINISTERED AS: an infusion, syrup or dietary item.

Dropwort, Hemlock water *Œnanthe crocata.*
COMMON NAME: horsebane, deadtongue, five-fingered root, water lovage, yellow water dropwort.
OCCURRENCE: common in ditches and watering places in England, particularly the southern counties.
PARTS USED: the roots.

MEDICINAL USES: the beneficial uses are few because this plant is virulently poisonous. A tincture is used to treat eruptive diseases of the skin, but with very small dosages and great caution. Poultices have been used to heal whitlows or ulcers. This wild plant is the most poisonous of our indigenous plants and many deaths have resulted from adults and children eating the leaves or roots mistakenly.
ADMINISTERED AS: tincture, poultice.

Dropwort, Water *Œnanthe phellandrium.*
COMMON NAME: fine-leaved water dropwort, water fennel, fine-leaved oenanthe, *Phellandrium aquaticum.*
OCCURRENCE: a common plant in ditches and water courses across Europe and Great Britain.
PARTS USED: the fruit, which yields an ethereal oil called water fennel oil. The main chemical in the oil is the terpene, phellandrene.
MEDICINAL USES: expectorant, alterative, diuretic. The fruits are used to ease chronic pectoral conditions like bronchitis, consumption and asthma and also works well against dyspepsia, intermittent fevers and ulcers. Applied externally, the root has been utilized as a remedy for haemorrhoids. When taken in too large amounts, causing an overdose, the fruit prompts vertigo, intoxication and other narcotic effects. If the root is eaten by mistake, it can prove fatal in the same manner as with HEMLOCK WATER DROPWORT (*Oenanthe crocata*) where stomach irritation, circulation failure, giddiness, convulsions and coma can occur.
ADMINISTERED AS: powdered fruit, tincture, essence.

Dwarf elder *Sanbucus ebulus.*
COMMON NAME: danewort, wallwort, ground elder, walewort, blood hilder.

OCCURRENCE: found in ruins and waste ground throughout Europe and the British Isles.
PARTS USED: the leaves, roots and berries.
MEDICINAL USES: expectorant, diuretic, diaphoretic, purgative. The leaves are used internally to ease inflammation of the kidney and liver, and have a healing effect when used as a poultice on swellings and contusions. Dwarf elder tea was prepared from the dried root, when ground, and is one of the finest remedies for dropsy. The fresh root, when used as a decoction, is a drastic purgative. Overall, the dwarf elder is much more drastic in action than the common ELDER (*Sambucus nigra*).
ADMINISTERED AS: fresh root, decoction, poultice, infusion.

Echinacea *Echinacea angustifolia.*
COMMON NAME: black sampson, coneflower, rudbeckia, *Brauneria pallida.*
OCCURRENCE: a native plant of the prairie regions of the United states, west of Ohio. Also cultivated in Britain.
PARTS USED: the dried root and the rhizome. The wood and the bark contain oil, resin and large quantities of inulin, inuloid, sucrose, betaine, two phytosterols and oleic, cerotic, linolic and palmatic fatty acids.
MEDICINAL USES: alterative, antiseptic. This herb is considered sacred by many North American Indian tribes including the Sioux Indians. The herb boosts the immune system and increases bodily resistance to infection. It is used for boils, septicaemia, cancer, syphilis and gangrene. Echinacea is of particular value in treating diphtheria, typhoid and other infectious fevers. The herb can be used to improve appetite and digestion and can ease haemorrhoids when administered via injection.
ADMINISTERED AS: poultice, infusion, injection, fresh herb.

Elder *Sambucus nigra.*
COMMON NAME: black elder, common elder, European elder, pipe tree, bore tree, bour tree.
OCCURRENCE: frequently seen in Europe and Great Britain.
PARTS USED: the bark, leaves, flowers and berries.
MEDICINAL USES: the bark is a strong purgative and in large doses is emetic. It has been used successfully in epilepsy, and a tincture of the young bark relieves asthmatic symptoms and croup in children. A tea made from elder roots was highly effective against dropsy. The leaves are used both fresh and dried and contain the alkaloid sambucine, a glucoside called sambunigrin, as well as hydrogenic acid, cane sugar and potassium nitrate amongst other compounds. The leaves are used in preparation of green elder ointment which is used domestically for bruises, haemorrhoids, sprains, chilblains and applied to wounds. Elder leaves have the same purgative effects as the bark (but produce more nausea) and have expectorant, diaphoretic and diuretic actions.

The elder flowers are either distilled into elderflower water or dried. The water is used in eye and skin lotions as it is mildly astringent and a gentle stimulant. When infused, the dried flowers make elderflower tea which is gently laxative, aperient and diaphoretic. It is an old-fashioned remedy for colds and influenza when taken hot, before bed. The tea is also recommended to be drunk before breakfast as a blood purifier. Elder flowers would also be made into a lotion or poultice for use on inflamed areas and into an ointment which was good on wounds, scalds and burns. The ointment was used on the battlefields in World War I and at home for chapped hands and chilblains.
ADMINISTERED AS: an infusion, tincture, ointment, syrup, lotion, distilled water, poultice and dried powder.

Elecampane *Inula helenium.*
COMMON NAME: scabwort, elf dock, wild sunflower, horseheal, velvet dock.
OCCURRENCE: a true native of southern England, temperate Europe and Asia, but cultivated for medicinal purposes in northern England and Scotland.
PARTS USED: the root. This plant is a rich source of the drug inulin.
MEDICINAL USES: diuretic, tonic, diaphoretic, expectorant, antiseptic, astringent, and gently stimulant. It is used principally in coughs, consumption and pulmonary complaints, e.g. bronchitis. It is also used in acute catarrhal afflictions, dyspepsia ans asthma. Internally, it is normally combined with other herbs, as a decoction. Applied externally, it is rubefacient, and used in treating sciatica and facial neuralgia. The active bitter principle in the herb, helenin, is a very powerful antiseptic and bacterial chemical. This has meant elecampane has been used against the Tubercle bacteria and in surgical dressings.
ADMINISTERED AS: powdered root, fluid extract, tincture, poultice, infusion.

Elm, Common *Ulmus campestris.*
COMMON NAME: field elm, ulmi cortex, broad-leaved elm.
OCCURRENCE: common in Britain, Europe, Asia and North Africa.
PARTS USED: the dried inner bark.
MEDICINAL USES: tonic, demulcent, astringent and diuretic. It was formerly employed as an antiscorbutic decoction recommended in skin diseases such as ringworm. Also used as a poultice to relieve pain from gout or rheumatism.
ADMINISTERED AS: tincture, fluid extract or tea.

Ephedra *Ephedra vulgaris.*
COMMON NAME: ephedrine, epitonin, mattuang.

OCCURRENCE: grows in west central China, southern Siberia and Japan.
PARTS USED: the stems, of which ephedrine is the active alkaloidal chemical.
MEDICINAL USES: nerve stimulant, antispasmodic. The herb resembles adrenaline in effect and it relieves swellings of the mucous membranes quickly. It has been used to treat asthma, hay fever and rheumatism as well as being a prophylactic drug to help low blood pressure in influenza or pneumonia.
ADMINISTERED AS: tablets, injection.

Ergot *Claviceps purpurea.*
COMMON NAME: ergot of rye, smut of rye, spurred rye, *Serale cornutum.*
OCCURRENCE: this herbal remedy is the fungal mycelium which grows parasitically on rye, wheat and other grasses.
PARTS USED: ergot contains two alkaloids—ergotoxine and ergotamine as the active chemicals.
MEDICINAL USES: emmenagogue, haemostatic, uterine, stimulant, and sedative. It is normally used as a muscle stimulant in menstrual disorders such as leucorrhoea and painful or lacking menstruation and can be used to stop internal haemorrhage with best results against uterine haemorrhage. It is used as a sedative in cases of delirium, asthma or hysteria and also acts as a galactogogue.
ADMINISTERED AS: extract, infusion, tincture, liquid extract.

Eryngo *Eryngicum campestre.*
COMMON NAME: sea holly, eringo, sea hulver, sea holme.
OCCURRENCE: found on sandy soils and seashores around England and the rest of Europe's coastline, but rare in Scotland.
PARTS USED: the root.
MEDICINAL USES: diaphoretic, diuretic, aromatic, stimulant, expec-

torant. It is good in dealing with coughs, consumption, paralysis and chronic nervous diseases. It has effective results against all diseases of the bladder, scorbutic complaints, jaundice and liver problems.
ADMINISTERED AS: decoction.

Eucalyptus *Eucalyptus globulus.*
COMMON NAME: blue gum tree, stringy bark tree.
OCCURRENCE: native to Australia and Tasmania; now introduced into North and South Africa, India and southern Europe.
PARTS USED: the oil distilled from the leaves. The oil contains eucalyptol, which is the important medically-active chemical.
MEDICINAL USES: antiseptic, antispasmodic, stimulant, aromatic. The oil is used as an antiseptic and stimulant gargle; it increases the action of the heart and is said to have some antimalarial properties. It is taken internally in pulmonary tuberculosis, scarlet, typhoid and intermittent fevers. The oil is used as an inhalant to clear catarrh and used externally to ease croup and throat troubles. However, in large doses it can irritate the kidneys, depress the nervous system and possibly stop respiration and breathing. Despite its harmless appearance, care should be used when administering the drug internally.
ADMINISTERED AS: distilled oil, emulsion.

Euphorbia *Euphorbia hirta.*
COMMON NAME: asthma-weed, catshair, *Euphorbia pilulifera.*
OCCURRENCE: grows in India and other tropical countries.
PARTS USED: the herb.
MEDICINAL USES: anti-asthmatic, pectoral. It is highly effective in treating paroxysmal asthma, coughs and bronchial and pulmonary disorders. In India it is used against syphilis.
ADMINISTERED AS: tincture, liquid extract.

Evening primrose *Oenothera biennis.*
COMMON NAME: tree primrose, sun drop.
OCCURRENCE: native to North America but has been naturalized to British and European gardens.
PARTS USED: the bark and leaves.
MEDICINAL USES: astringent, sedative. The drug from this herb is not extensively used but has been of benefit in treating gastro-intestinal disorders, dyspepsia, liver torpor and in female problems in association with pelvic illness. It has also been successfully used in whooping cough and spasmodic asthma.
ADMINISTERED AS: liquid extract.

Eyebright *Euphrasia officinalis.*
COMMON NAME: euphrasia.
OCCURRENCE: a wild plant growing in meadows and grasslands in England and Europe.
PARTS USED: the herb. This plant contains various chemicals including euphrasia-tannin, mannite and glucose.
MEDICINAL USES: slightly tonic and astringent. As its name suggests, eyebright is recommended in treating diseases of the sight, weak eyes, etc. It is generally used as an infusion in water or milk and is combined in a lotion with GOLDEN SEAL, the pairing said to be highly effective.
ADMINISTERED AS: infusion, ointment or expressed juice.

Fennel *Foeniculum vulgare.*
COMMON NAME: hinojo, fenkel, sweet fennel, wild fennel.
OCCURRENCE: found wild in most areas of temperate Europe and generally considered indigenous to the shores of the Mediterranean. It is cultivated for medicinal benefit in France, Russia, India and Persia.
PARTS USED: the seeds, leaves and roots. The roots are rarely used

in herbal medicine today. The essential oil is separated by distillation with water. Fennel oil varies widely in quality and composition dependent upon where and under what conditions the fennel was grown.

MEDICINAL USES: aromatic, stimulant, carminative and stomachic. The herb is principally used with purgatives to allay their tendency to griping, and the seeds form an ingredient of the compound liquorice powder. Fennel water also acts in a similar manner to DILL water in correcting infant flatulence.

ADMINISTERED AS: fluid extract, distilled water, essential oil.

Fenugreek *Trigonella foenum-graecum.*

COMMON NAME: bird's foot, Greek hay-seed.

OCCURRENCE: indigenous to eastern Mediterranean countries, but is cultivated in India, Africa and England.

PARTS USED: the seeds. These contain mucilage, two alkaloids trigonelline and choline—phosphates, lecithin and nucleoalbumin.

MEDICINAL USES: a preparation where seeds are soaked in water until they swell and form a thick paste is used to prevent fevers, is comforting to the stomach and has been utilized for diabetes. Alcoholic tinctures are used to prepare emollient cream, ointments and plasters while the mucilage is used externally as a poultice for skin infections such as abscesses, boils and carbuncles. It is also good at relieving rickets, anaemia and scrofula, while, combined with the normal dosage of conventional medicine e.g insulin, it is helpful in gout, diabetes and neurasthenia. It is widely used as a flavouring for both human and cattle feed.

ADMINISTERED AS: poultice, ointment, infusion or tincture.

Feverfew *Chrysanthemum parthenium.*

COMMON NAME: featherfew, featherfoil, flirtwort, bachelor's buttons, pyrethrum parthenium.

OCCURRENCE: a wild hedgerow plant found in many areas of Europe and Great Britain.
PARTS USED: the herb.
MEDICINAL USES: aperient, carminative, bitter, stimulant, emmenagogue. It is employed in hysterical complaints, nervousness and low spirits as a general tonic. A decoction is made and is useful in easing coughs, wheezing and difficult breathing. Earache was relieved by a cold infusion while a tincture of feverfew eased the pain and swelling caused after insect or vermin bites. The herb was planted around dwellings to purify the atmosphere and ward off disease. Today, it is used to prevent or ease migraines or headaches.
ADMINISTERED AS: warm or cold infusion, poultice, tincture, decoction.

Fig *Ficus carica.*
COMMON NAME: common fig.
OCCURRENCE: indigenous to Persia, Asia Minor and Syria, but cultivated in most of the Mediterranean countries and England.
PARTS USED: the fleshy inflorescence (so-called fruit).
MEDICINAL USES: nutritive, emollient, demulcent, laxative. It is normally utilized in laxative confections and syrups with SENNA and carminatives. Demulcent decoctions are prepared from figs and are used in treating catarrhal afflictions of the nose and throat. Roasted figs, when split open, are used as a poultice to gumboils, dental abscesses, boils and carbuncles. The fruit is used both fresh and dried.
ADMINISTERED AS: poultice, syrup, decoction.

Figwort *Scrophularia nodosa.*
COMMON NAME: rose noble, throatwort, carpenter's square, kernelwort, scrofula plant.

OCCURRENCE: a wild plant of Great Britain and Europe.
PARTS USED: the herb.
MEDICINAL USES: diuretic, anodyne, depurative. Due to this herb's beneficial action on skin abscesses, eruptions and wounds, it has been termed the scrofula plant. The fresh leaves are used as a poultice on sprains, swellings, inflammation, wounds, gangrene and scrofulous sores to great effect.
ADMINISTERED AS: decoction, fresh leaves, dried herb, ointment and fluid extract.

Fireweed *Erechtites hieracifolia* or *Cineraria caradensis*.
COMMON NAME: *Senecio hieracifolius*.
OCCURRENCE: a common weed found in Newfoundland and Canada and south to South America.
PARTS USED: the herb, and the oil of erechtites distilled from the herb. The oil is composed of various terpene chemicals.
MEDICINAL USES: astringent, alterative, tonic, cathartic, emetic. Taken internally, it is good for eczema, diarrhoea, haemorrhages and sore throats. It has also been used for colic, spasms, hiccoughs, dysentery and haemorrhoids. When used externally, the oil gives great relief to gout, rheumatism and sciatica.
ADMINISTERED AS: distilled oil in capsules or emulsion, tincture.

Flax *Linum usitatissimum*.
COMMON NAME: linseed.
OCCURRENCE: grows in most temperate and tropical countries.
PARTS USED: the seeds and oil expressed from the seeds, a cake remains which can be ground up to form linseed meal.
MEDICINAL USES: emollient, demulcent, pectoral. A poultice of linseed meal, either alone or with mustard, is effective in relieving pain and irritation from boils, ulcers, inflamed areas and abscesses. Flax is normally utilized as an addition to cough medicines, while

linseed oil is sometimes given as a laxative or to remove gravel and stones. When mixed with LIME water the oil is excellent on burns and scalds.

ADMINISTERED AS: essential oil, ground seed coats (meal), infusion, syrup and poultice.

Foxglove *Digitalis purpurea.*

COMMON NAME: witch's gloves, dead men's bells, fairy's glove, gloves of Our Lady, bloody fingers, virgin's glove, fairy caps, folk's glove, fairy thimbles, fair women's plant.

OCCURRENCE: indigenous and widely distributed throughout Great Britain and Europe.

PARTS USED: the leaves, which contain four important glucosides—digitoxin, digitalin, digitalein and digitonin—of which the first three listed are cardiac stimulants.

MEDICINAL USES: cardiac tonic, sedative, diuretic. Administering digitalis increases the activity of all forms of muscle tissue, particularly the heart and arterioles. It causes a very high rise in blood pressure and the pulse is slowed and becomes regular. Digitalis causes the heart to contract in size, allowing increased blood flow and nutrient delivery to the organ. It also acts on the kidneys and is a good remedy for dropsy, particularly when it is connected with cardiac problems. The drug has benefits in treating internal haemorrhage, epilepsy, inflammatory diseases and delirium tremens. Digitalis has a cumulative action whereby it is liable to accumulate in the body and then have poisonous effects. It should only be used under medical advice. Digitalis is an excellent antidote in ACONITE poisoning when given as a hypodermic injection.

ADMINISTERED AS: tincture, infusion, powdered leaves, solid extract, injection.

Fringe tree *Chionanthus virginica.*
COMMON NAME: old man's beard, snowdrop tree, poison ash, fringe tree bark, chionanthus.
OCCURRENCE: a small tree, native to the southern United States.
PARTS USED: the dried bark of the root which is thought to contain saponin and a glucoside.
MEDICINAL USES: aperient, diuretic, alterative, tonic. The root is used in typhoid, intermittent or bilious fevers, in liver complaints, jaundice and gallstones. It is taken in conjunction with ANEMONE PULSATILLA and other herbs for women's complaints. Also used as a poultice on wounds and inflammations.
ADMINISTERED AS: infusion, fluid extract.

Frostwort *Helianthemum canadense.*
COMMON NAME: cistus, frostweed, frostplant, rock rose, *Cistus canadensis, Lechea Major, Canadisches Sonnenroschen, Helianthemum ramultoflorum, H. rosmarinifolium, H. michauxii, H. Coprymbosum, Hetraneris canadensis.*
OCCURRENCE: grows in the eastern United States, Great Britain and Europe.
PARTS USED: the dried herb. The main chemical components are a volatile oil, wax, tannin, fatty oil, chlorophyll, gum, inorganic salts and a glucoside.
MEDICINAL USES: antiscrofulous, astringent, alterative, tonic. The herb has a long history of use for diarrhoea, ulcerations, eye complaints, secondary syphilis and any conditions arising from scrofula. It has been beneficial as a poultice for tumours and ulcers and as a gargle in scarlatina. An overdose of the drug is possible and causes nausea and vomiting.
ADMINISTERED AS: liquid extract.

Fumitory *Fumaria officinalis.*
COMMON NAME: earth smoke, beggary, fumus, vapor, nidor, fumus terrae, fumiterry, scheiteregi, taubenkropp, kaphnos, wax dolls.
OCCURRENCE: a common weed plant in Great Britain and Europe, which has been naturalized into North America; originally from Asia and Greece.
PARTS USED: the herb and the expressed juice and fluid extract derived from it.
MEDICINAL USES: weak tonic, diaphoretic, diuretic, aperient. This herb is valuable in all internal obstructions, particularly those of the liver and stomach and is also of benefit in scorbutic afflictions and skin eruptions including leprosy. It is the preferred herb to purify the blood in France and Germany, and in some areas it is smoked as tobacco. It was said to aid removal of skin blemishes and freckles and was also used to ease dyspepsia and headaches.
ADMINISTERED AS: expressed juice, essence, syrup, distilled water, decoction, dried herb, several different tinctures, powdered seed.

Gale, Sweet *Myrica gale.*
COMMON NAME: bayberry, English bog myrtle, Dutch myrtle, gale palustris.
OCCURRENCE: a bushy shrub found in higher latitudes of the northern hemisphere; abundant in Scottish moors and bogs.
PARTS USED: the shrub.
MEDICINAL USES: aromatic, astringent. The leaves have been used as an emmenagogue and an abortifacient (induces abortion or miscarriage).
ADMINISTERED AS: dried leaves and infusion.

Garlic *Allium sativum.*
COMMON NAME: poor man's treacle.
OCCURRENCE: cultivated throughout Europe since antiquity.

PARTS USED: the bulb.
MEDICINAL USES: antiseptic, diaphoretic, diuretic, expectorant, stimulant. It may be externally applied as ointment, lotion, antiseptic or as a poultice. Syrup of garlic is very good for asthma, coughs, difficulty in breathing and chronic bronchitis, while fresh juice has been used to ease tubercular consumption. The essential oil is commonly taken as a supplement in the form of gelatine capsules. Several species of wild garlic are utilized for both medicinal and dietary purposes.
ADMINISTERED AS: expressed juice, syrup, tincture, essential oil, poultice, lotion and ointment.

Gelsemium *Gelsemium sempervirens.*
COMMON NAME: yellow jasmine, *Gelsemium nitridum*, false jasmine, wild woodbine, Carolina jasmine.
OCCURRENCE: a native North American plant found along the sea coast from Virginia, to southern Florida and Mexico.
PARTS USED: the root which contains two alkaloids—gelsemium and gelsemine, as well as gelsemic acid, a volatile oil, resin and starch.
MEDICINAL USES: antispasmodic, arterial sedative, diaphoretic, febrifuge. Used in small doses to treat neuralgic pains, muscular irritability, nervous excitement and hysteria while its antispasmodic qualities aid asthma, whooping cough, croup and convulsions with great success. It relaxes all muscles and acts on the whole body to remove all sense of pain. The root is very good against bowel inflammation, diarrhoea, dysentery, toothache, chorea, epilepsy, insomnia and headaches due to sickness or alcohol consumption. The drug also benefits acute rheumatism, pleurisy, pneumonia, bronchitis, typhoid fever and pelvic disorders in women. This drug is poisonous and so should be administered in small doses, with very careful monitoring of the patient. Death

occurs due to the action of the drug on nervous control of the respiratory system, and can occur very quickly after taking the drug—between one and seven hours after ingestion. Treatment of gelsemium poisoning must be rapid with evacuation of the stomach, artificial respiration and the use of atropine, BELLADONNA (*Atropa belladonna*); strychnine, NUX VOMICA (*Strychnos nux-vomica*); or digitalis, FOXGLOVE (*Digitalis purpurea*) to maintain action of the heart being recommended.
ADMINISTERED AS: tincture, solid extract, infusion.

Gentian, Yellow *Gentiana lutea.*
OCCURRENCE: native to alpine regions of central and southern Europe.
PARTS USED: the root. The dried root contains gentian, gentiamarin, bitter glucosides, gentianic acid and various sugars. The fresh root also contains gentiopicrin, another bitter glucoside.
MEDICINAL USES: bitter tonic, stomachic, febrifuge, emmenagogue, anthelmintic and antiseptic. This drug is probably the most effective bitter tonic of use in exhaustion from chronic disease, general debility, weakness of the digestive organs and lack of appetite. It acts to strengthen the whole body and is a very good tonic to combine with purgative drugs in order to temper their debilitating effects. Yellow gentian is useful in many dyspeptic complaints, hysteria, female weakness, intermittent fevers and jaundice. The roots have also been used to make an alcoholic beverage in Germany and Switzerland.
ADMINISTERED AS: infusion, tincture, solid extract, fluid extract.

Germander, Wall *Teucrium chamaedys.*
COMMON NAME: petit chêne, chasse fièvre.
OCCURRENCE: a native of many parts of Europe, the Greek Islands and Syria but is an escape from garden cultivation in England.

PARTS USED: the whole herb, dried.
MEDICINAL USES: stimulant, tonic, diaphoretic, diuretic, aperient. Germander has a reputation as a specific cure for gout, dating back to the sixteenth century. It has been used as a tonic in treating intermittent fevers and uterine obstructions and a decoction of the fresh herb is good against asthmatic afflictions and coughs. The expressed juice is taken for obstructions of the viscera, while the herb has also been used for jaundice, as a vermifuge, ulcers, continual headache and cramps.
ADMINISTERED AS: expressed juice, poultice, decoction, powdered seeds.

Ginger *Zingiber officinale*.
OCCURRENCE: a native of Asia, it is now cultivated in the West Indies, Jamaica and Africa.
PARTS USED: the root, which contains volatile oil, two resins, gum, starch, lignin, acetic acid and asmazone as well as several unidentified compounds.
MEDICINAL USES: stimulant, carminative, expectorant. A valuable herb in dyspepsia, flatulent colic, alcoholic gastritis and diarrhoea. Ginger tea is taken to relieve the effects of cold temperatures including triggering normal menstruation patterns in women. Ginger is also used to flavour bitter infusions, cough mixtures or syrups.

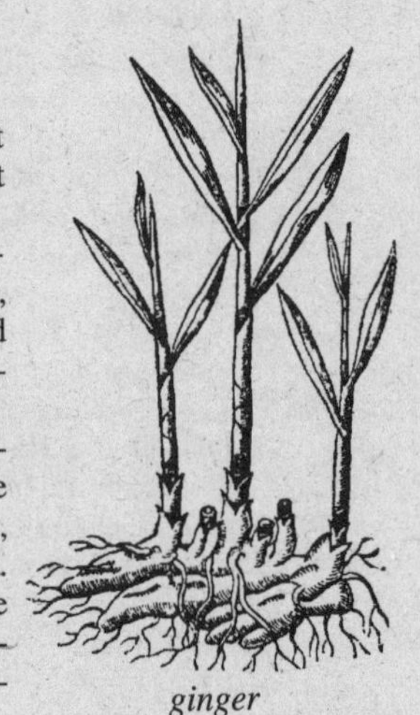
ginger

ADMINISTERED AS: infusion, fluid extract, tincture and syrup.

Ginseng *Panax quinquefolium.*
COMMON NAME: *Aralia quinquefolia*, five fingers, tartar root, red berry, man's health, panax, pannag.
OCCURRENCE: native to certain areas of China, eastern Asia and North America. It is largely cultivated in China, Korea and Japan.
PARTS USED: the root which contains a large quantity of gum, resin, volatile oil and the peculiar sweetish compound, panaquilon.
MEDICINAL USES: mild stomachic, tonic, stimulant. The generic name, *panax*, is derived from the Greek for panacea meaning "all-healing." The name ginseng is said to mean "the wonder of the world" and the Chinese consider this herb a sovereign remedy in all diseases. It is good in dyspepsia, vomiting and nervous disorders, consumption and exhaustion. In the West, it is used to treat loss of appetite, stomach and digestive problems, possibly arising from nervous and mental exhaustion. Ginseng is considered to work well against fatigue, old age and its infirmities and to help convalescents recover their health. In healthy people, the drug is said to increase vitality, cure pulmonary complaints and tumours and increase life expectancy. It was also used by the native American Indians for similar problems.
ADMINISTERED AS: tincture, decoction, capsules.

Gladwyn *Iris foetidissina.*
COMMON NAME: stinking gladwyn, gladwin, gladwine, stinking gladdon, spurgewort, spurge plant, roast beef plant.
OCCURRENCE: found in woods and shady parts in southern England.
PARTS USED: the root.
MEDICINAL USES: antispasmodic, cathartic, anodyne. A decoction acts as a strong purge; has been used as an emmenagogue and for removing eruptions. The dried powdered root can be of benefit in hysterical disorders, fainting, nervous problems and to relieve cramps and

pain. Taken both internally and as an external poultice, this is an excellent herb to remedy scrofula. The use of this herbal remedy can be dated back to the fourth century before Christ.
ADMINISTERED AS: decoction, dried root, infusion.

Globe flower *Trollius europaeus.*
COMMON NAME: globe trollius, boule d'or, European globe flower, globe rananculus, globe crow-foot, luchen-gowans.
OCCURRENCE: a native European plant found in moist woods and mountain pastures.
PARTS USED: the whole plant, fresh.
MEDICINAL USES: currently this plant is not used to treat many diseases and it has properties which would benefit from further investigation. It has been used in Russia to treat obstinate scorbutic disorders.

Golden rod *Solidago virgaurea.*
COMMON NAME: verge d'or, solidago, goldruthe, woundwort, Aaron's rod.
OCCURRENCE: normally found wild in woods in Britain, Europe, central Asia and North America but it is also a common garden plant.
PARTS USED: the leaves contain tannin, with some bitter and astringent chemicals which are unknown.
MEDICINAL USES: aromatic, stimulant, carminative. This herb is astringent and diuretic and is highly effective in curing gravel and urinary stones. It aids weak digestion, stops sickness and is very good against diphtheria. As a warm infusion it is a good diaphoretic drug and is used as such to help painful menstruation and amenorrhoea (absence or stopping of menstrual periods).
ADMINISTERED AS: fluid extract, infusion, spray.

Golden seal *Hydrastis canadensis.*
COMMON NAME: orange root, yellow root, yellow puccoon, ground raspberry, wild curcuma, tumeric root, Indian root, eyebalm, Indian paint, jaundice root, warnera, eye root.
OCCURRENCE: a native plant of Canada and eastern United States.
PARTS USED: the rhizome which contains the alkaloids berberine, hydastine and canadine, as well as resin, albumin, starch, fatty matter, sugar, lignin and volatile oil.
MEDICINAL USES: tonic, stomachic, laxative, alterative, detergent. Native American Indians use this plant as a source of yellow dye for clothing and weapons and also as a remedy for sore eyes, general ulceration and disordered digestion. The herb has a special action on the mucous membranes of the body, making it an excellent remedy for catarrh, dyspepsia, gastric catarrh, loss of appetite and liver problems. Given as a tonic, the root is highly effective in easing constipation and is very good at stopping sickness and vomiting. Chronic inflammation of the colon and rectum can be treated by an injection of golden seal, as can haemorrhoids. When taken as an infusion, it may cure night-sweats and passive bleeding from the pelvic tissues. In large doses, *Hydrastis* is very poisonous.
ADMINISTERED AS: injection, infusion, tincture, lotion, fluid extract, dried powdered root, solid extract.

Gooseberry *Ribes grossularia.*
COMMON NAME: fea, feverberry, feabes, carberry, groseille, groset, groser, krusbaar, dewberries, goosegogs, honeyblobs, feaberry.
OCCURRENCE: a well-known shrub native to central and northern Europe, especially Great Britain.
PARTS USED: the fruit and leaves, which contain citric acid, sugar, various minerals and pectose.
MEDICINAL USES: the expressed juice is said to be a cure for all

inflammations. The acid red fruit is made into a light jelly which is good for sedentary and bilious complaints as well as in cases of excess body fluid. An infusion of dried leaves is effective in treating gravel and is a useful tonic for menstruating young girls. In the Highlands of Scotland, the prickles were used as charms to remove warts and styes.
ADMINISTERED AS: an infusion, expressed juice, dietary item.

Goutwort *Aegopodium podagraria.*
COMMON NAME: goutweed, goutherb, ashweed, Jack-jump-about, herb gerard, English masterwort, pigweed, eltroot, ground elder, bishops elder, white ash, ground ash, weyl ash, bishopsweed.
OCCURRENCE: a weed plant of Europe, Great Britain and Russian Asia.
PARTS USED: the herb.
MEDICINAL USES: diuretic and sedative. Taken internally for aching joints, gouty and sciatic pain and as an external poultice for inflamed areas. It was thought that carrying some of the herb in a pocket would prevent an attack of gout developing.
ADMINISTERED AS: poultice, liquid extract.

Groundsel *Senecio vulgaris.*
COMMON NAME: common groundsel, grundy, swallow, ground glutton, simson, sention, grounsel.
OCCURRENCE: very common weed throughout Europe and Russian Asia.
PARTS USED: the whole herb and fresh plant. The plant contains senecin and seniocine.
MEDICINAL USES: diaphoretic, anti scorbutic, purgative, diuretic, anthelmintic. It is good for sickness of the stomach, used as a purgative in a weak infusion and as an emetic when in a strong infusion. This infusion removes bilious trouble and lowers body temperature.

A poultice of groundsel is used warm on boils but nursing mothers have cold poultices as a coolant on swollen inflamed or hardened breasts. If boiling water is poured on to the fresh plant, the resulting liquid is a pleasant swab for the skin and helps soften chapped hands.
ADMINISTERED AS: infusion, poultice lotion.

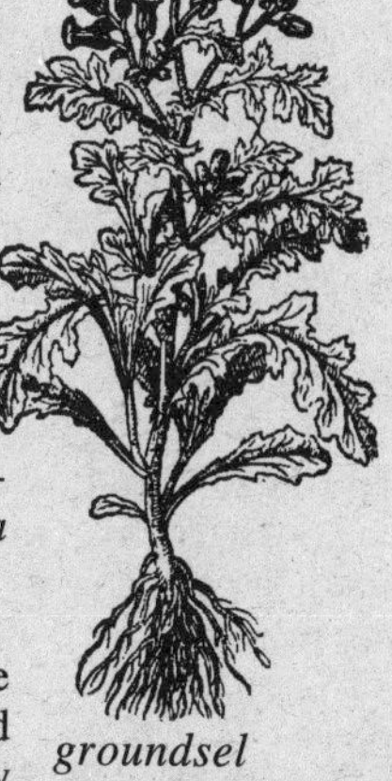
groundsel

Guarana *Paullinia cupara.*
COMMON NAME: paullina, guarana bread, Brazilian cocoa, uabano, uaranzeiro, *Paullina sorbilis*.
OCCURRENCE: native to Brazil and Uruguay.
PARTS USED: the prepared seed, crushed. The seeds are shelled, roasted for six hours and shaken until their outer shell comes off. They are ground to a fine powder, made into a dough with water and formed into cylinders which are dried in the sun or over a fire. The seed preparation is eaten with water by the native people. The roasted seeds contain caffeine, tannic acid, catechutannic acid, starch and a fixed oil.
MEDICINAL USES: nervine, tonic, stimulant, aphrodisiac, febrifuge, slightly narcotic. It is used in mild forms of diarrhoea or leucorrhoea and also for headaches, in particular those linked to the menstrual cycle. guarana stimulates the brain after mental exertion, or after fatigue or exhaustion due to hot temperatures. It may also have diuretic effects where it can help rheumatism, lumbago and bowel complaints. The drug is similar to that of COCA or COFFEE.
ADMINISTERED AS: powder, fluid extract, tincture.

Hair-cap moss *Polytrichium juniperum.*
COMMON NAME: bear's bed, robin's eye, ground moss, golden maidenhair, female fern herb, robinsrye, rockbrake herb.
OCCURRENCE: found in woods and hedges across Europe and Britain.
PARTS USED: the whole plant.
MEDICINAL USES: powerful diuretic. It is a very important remedy in dropsy, urinary obstructions, gravel and suppression of urine. The herb does not cause nausea and is frequently combined with BROOM or CARROT for best effects.
ADMINISTERED AS: infusion.

Hawthorn *Crataegus oxyacantha.*
COMMON NAME: may, mayblossom, quick, thorn, whitethorn, haw, hazels, gazels, halves, hagthorn, ladies meat, bread and cheese tree, maybush.
OCCURRENCE: a familiar tree in Great Britain, Europe, North Africa and Western Asia.
PARTS USED: the dried fruits.which contain the chemical amyddalin.
MEDICINAL USES: cardiac, diuretic, astringent, tonic. Mainly used as a cardiac tonic in organic and functional heart problems, e.g. hypertrophy, dyspnoea, heart oppression. A decoction of the flowers and berries is good at curing sore throats, and is utilized as a diuretic in dropsy and kidney disorders.
ADMINISTERED AS: liquid extract, decoction.

Heartease *Viola tricolor.*
COMMON NAME: wild pansy, love-lies-bleeding, loving idol, call-me-to-you, three-faces-under-a-hood, godfathers and godmothers, pink-eyed-John, flower o'luce, Jack-jump-up-and-kiss-me.
OCCURRENCE: abundant all over Great Britain, in cornfields, gardens, waste ground and hedge banks. It is also distributed through Arctic Europe, North Africa, Siberia and North India.

PARTS USED: the whole herb, fresh and dried. The active chemicals within the plant include violine, mucilage, resin, salicylic acid and sugar.
MEDICINAL USES: diaphoretic and diuretic. It was formerly held in high regard as a remedy for epilepsy, asthma and catarrhal infections. It has been utilized in blood disorders and heart diseases, while a decoction of the flowers was recommended for skin diseases. In America, they use heartease as an ointment or poultice in eczema, and it is taken internally for bronchitis. People on the continent have used *Viola tricolor* for its mucilaginous, demulcent and expectorant qualities.
ADMINISTERED AS: decoction, ointment, poultice and tincture.

Hedge-hyssop *Gratiola officinalis.*
OCCURRENCE: a perennial plant, native to southern Europe and found wild in damp areas in Great Britain.
PARTS USED: the root and herb. The plant contains the glucosides gratiolin and gratiosolin.
MEDICINAL USES: diuretic, cathartic, emetic. Recommended in scrofula, chronic liver complaints and enlargement of the spleen. It is also utilized in relieving dropsy and as a vermifuge.
ADMINISTERED AS: an infusion of powdered root.

Hellebore, Black *Helleborus niger.*
COMMON NAME: Christe herbe, Christmas rose, melampodium.
OCCURRENCE: a native of the mountains in central and southern Europe, Greece and Asia minor, but found in Britain as a garden plant.
PARTS USED: the rhizome and root. The plant has two glucosides within it, helleborin and helleborcin, both of which are powerful poisons.
MEDICINAL USES: the drug has drastic purgative, emmenagogue and

anthelmintic properties, but is a violent narcotic. It is of value in treating nervous disorders, hysteria and melancholia and was previously used in dropsy and amenorrhoea. Given externally, the fresh root is violently irritant. The drug must be administered with great care.
ADMINISTERED AS: fluid extract, tincture, solid extract, powdered root or decoction.

Hemlock *Conium maculatum.*
COMMON NAME: herb bennet, spotted conebane, musquash root, beaver poison, poison hemlock, poison parsley, spotted hemlock, vex, vecksies.
OCCURRENCE: common in hedges, meadows, waste ground and stream banks throughout Europe and is also found in temperate Asia and North Africa.
PARTS USED: the leaves, fruits and seeds. The most important constituent of hemlock leaves is the alkaloid coniine, which is poison-ous, with a disagreeable odour. Other alkaloids in the plant include methyl-coniine, conhydrine, pseudoconhydrine, ethyl piperidine.
MEDICINAL USES: sedative, antispasmodic, anodyne. The drug acts on the centres of motion and causes paralysis and so it is used to remedy undue nervous motor excitability, e.g. teething, cramp and muscle spasms of the larynx and gullet. When inhaled, hemlock is said to be good in relieving coughs, bronchitis, whooping cough and asthma. The method of action of *Conium* means it is directly antagonistic to the effects of strychnine, from NUX VOMICA (*Strychnos nux-vomica*), and hence it is used as an antidote to strychnine poisoning and similar poisons. Hemlock has to be administered with care as narcotic poisoning may result from internal application and overdoses induce paralysis, with loss of speech and depression of respiratory function leading to death. Antidotes

to hemlock poisoning are tannic acid, stimulants, e.g. COFFEE, MUSTARD and CASTOR OIL.
ADMINISTERED AS: powdered leaves, fluid extract, tincture, expressed juice of the leaves and solid extract.

Henbane *Hyoscyamus niger.*
COMMON NAME: hyoscyamus, hog's bean, Jupiter's-bean, symphonica, cassilata, cassilago, deus caballinus.
OCCURRENCE: native to central and southern Europe and western Asia and was introduced to Great Britain, North America and Brazil where it is found on waste ground, ditches and near old buildings.
PARTS USED: the fresh leaves and flowering tops. The chief constituents of henbane leaves are the alkaloids hyoscyamine, atropine and hyoscine. The leaves also contain a bitter principle called hyoscytricin, choline, mucilage, calcium oxalate, potassium nitrate and fixed oil.
MEDICINAL USES: antispasmodic, hypnotic, mild diuretic, mydriatic, anodyne, sedative. The herb has a milder narcotic effect than BELLADONNA or STRAMONIUM and is utilized to lessen muscle spasms, reduce pain and can stop nervous irritation. It is used in cystitis, irritable bladder, hysteria, irritable cough, asthma, gastric ulcers and chronic gastric catarrh. When taken in small doses repeated over time, Henbane tranquillizes people affected by severe nervous irritability, enabling them to sleep without adversely affecting the digestive organs or causing headaches, which opium has the tendency to do. Thus, henbane is given to people with insomnia and to children, to which opium cannot be given. The fresh leaves of henbane can be used as a poultice to relieve local pain from gout, neuralgia, cancerous ulcers, sores and swellings. The solid extract of the drug is used to produce suppositories which are used to relieve the pain of haemorrhoids. Henbane

is poisonous and should never be used except under medical advice.
ADMINISTERED AS: powdered leaves, tincture, fluid extract, expressed juice, solid extract, suppositories.

Holly *Ilex aquifolium.*
COMMON NAME: holm, hulver bush, hulm, holme chase, holy tree, Christ's thorn.
OCCURRENCE: native to central and southern Europe and grows freely in Great Britain.
PARTS USED: the leaves, berries and bark.
MEDICINAL USES: diaphoretic, febrifuge, cathartic, tonic. Infused holly leaves are used in catarrh, pleurisy and formerly against smallpox. Also in intermittent fevers and rheumatism where the alkaloid ilicin works to good effect. Juice expressed from fresh holly leaves is effective against jaundice. The berries have different properties and are violently emetic and purgative, but they have been utilized in dropsy and as a powder to check bleeding. Holly leaves have been utilized as a tea substitute.
ADMINISTERED AS: infusion of leaves, juice, whole or powdered berries.

Honeysuckle *Lonicera caprifolium.*
COMMON NAME: Dutch honeysuckle, goat's leaf, perfoliate honeysuckle.
OCCURRENCE: grows freely in Europe, Great Britain and throughout the northern temperate zone.
PARTS USED: the dried flowers and leaves
MEDICINAL USES: expectorant, laxative. A syrup made of the flowers is used for respiratory diseases and asthma. A decoction of the leaves is laxative and is also good against diseases of the liver and spleen, and in gargles.
ADMINISTERED AS: syrup, decoction.

Hops *Humulus lupulus.*

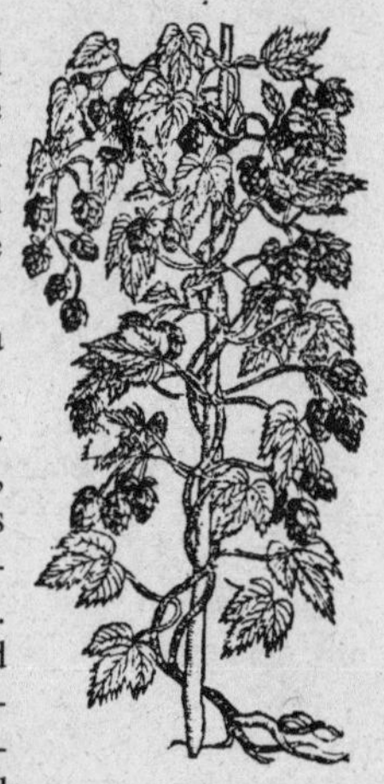

hops

OCCURRENCE: a native British plant, found wild in hedges and woods from Yorkshire southward. It is considered an introduced species to Scotland but is also found in most countries of the northern temperate zone.

PARTS USED: the flowers, which contain a volatile oil, two bitter principles—lupamaric acid, lupalinic acid- and tannin.

MEDICINAL USES: tonic, nervine, diuretic, anodyne, aromatic. The volatile oil has sedative and soporific effects while the bitter principles are stomachic and tonic. Hops are used to promote the appetite and enhance sleep. An infusion is very effective in heart disease, fits, neuralgia, indigestion, jaundice, nervous disorders and stomach or liver problems. Hop juice is a blood cleanser and is very effective in remedying calculus problems. As an external application, hops are used with CHAMOMILE heads as an infusion to reduce painful swellings or inflammation and bruises. This combination may also be used as a poultice.

ADMINISTERED AS: an infusion, tincture, poultice, expressed juice or tea.

Horehound *Marrubium vulgare.*

COMMON NAME: hoarhound, white horehound.

OCCURRENCE: indigenous to Britain and found all over Europe.

PARTS USED: the herb, which contains the bitter principle marrubium, volatile oil, tannin sugar and resin.

MEDICINAL USES: tonic, expectorant, pectoral, diuretic. It is prob-

ably the most popular pectoral herbal remedy. Very valuable in coughs, asthma, consumption and pulmonary complaints. For children, it is given as a syrup to ease croup, stomach upsets and as a tonic. Taken in large doses, Horehound is a gentle purgative and the powdered leaves have been used as a vermifuge. A tea of the herb is excellent for colds. A sweetmeat candy and an ale is also made from horehound.
ADMINISTERED AS: syrup, infusion, tea, powdered leaves, ointment, expressed juice.

Horsemint, American *Monarda punctata.*
OCCURRENCE: native to North America and was introduced into England 1714.
PARTS USED: the herb produces a volatile oil which is composed of thymol and higher oxygenated compounds.
MEDICINAL USES: rubefacient, stimulant, carminative, diuretic. It is used as an infusion for flatulent colic, sickness and urinary disorders and has diaphoretic and emmenagogue actions also. It is principally used externally wherever a rubefacient is required, e.g. chronic rheumatism.
ADMINISTERED AS: a volatile oil.

Horseradish *Cochlearia armoracia.*
COMMON NAME: mountain radish, great raifort, red cole, *Armoracia rusticara.*
OCCURRENCE: cultivated in the British Isles for centuries. The place of origin is unknown.
PARTS USED: the root which contains the glucoside sinigrin, vitamin C, aspargin and resin.
MEDICINAL USES: stimulant, aperient, rubefacient, diuretic, antiseptic, diaphoretic. Horseradish is a powerful stimulant of the digestive organs, and it acts on lung and urinary infections clearing

them away. The herb is a very strong diuretic and as such is used to ease dropsy, gravel and calculus, as well as being taken internally for gout and rheumatism. A poultice can be made from the fresh root and applied to rheumatic joints, chilblains and to ease facial neuralgia. Horseradish juice, when diluted with vinegar and glycerine, was used in children's whooping cough and to relieve hoarseness of the throat. An infusion of the root in urine was stimulating to the entire nervous system and promoted perspiration, while it was also used to expel worms in children. Care should be taken when using this herb because over-use of horseradish can blister the skin and is not suitable for people with thyroid troubles.

ADMINISTERED AS: infusion, syrup, expressed juice, fluid extract.

Horsetail *Equisetum arvense.*

COMMON NAME: mare's tail, shave-grass, bottlebrush, paddock-pipes, Dutch rushes, pewterwort.

OCCURRENCE: native to Great Britain and distributed through temperate northern regions.

PARTS USED: the herb which is composed of silica, saponin, flavonoids, tannin and traces of alkaloids—nicotine, palustrine and palustrinine.

MEDICINAL USES: diuretic, astringent. Due to the herb's rich store of minerals, horsetail is given for anaemia and general debility and can also work to encourage the absorption and efficient use of calcium by the body, helping prevent fatty deposits forming in the arteries (arteriosclerosis). It helps stop bleeding and hence is good for stomach ulcers and haemorrhage as well as easing dropsy, gravel, cystitis and inflamed prostate glands due to its astringent qualities. The herb can be of benefit in the treatment of bed-wetting in children.

ADMINISTERED AS: infusion, dried herb, syrup.

Hound's tongue *Cynoglossum officinale.*
COMMON NAME: dog's tongue, *Lindefolia spectabilis.*
OCCURRENCE: a common plant in Switzerland and Germany; occasionally found in Great Britain.
PARTS USED: the herb.
MEDICINAL USES: anodyne, demulcent, astringent. Used as pills or as a decoction for colds, coughs, catarrh, diarrhoea and dysentery. Administered both internally and externally to soothe the digestive organs and haemorrhoids.
ADMINISTERED AS: decoction, pills, ointment.

Houseleek *Sempervivum tectorum.*
COMMON NAME: Jupiter's eye, Thor's beard, bullock's eye, sengreen, ayron, ayegreen.
OCCURRENCE: native to the mountains of central and southern Europe and the Greek islands but introduced to Britain many centuries ago.
PARTS USED: the fresh leaves.
MEDICINAL USES: refrigerant, astringent, diuretic. The bruised fresh leaves or its expressed juice are often applied as a poultice to burns, scalds, bumps, scrofulous ulcers and general skin inflammation. The juice is a cure for warts and corns. In large doses, houseleek juice is emetic and purgative. The plant was supposed to guard where it grew against fire, lightning and sorcery, hence it was grown on house roofs.

Hydrangea *Hydrangea aborescens.*
COMMON NAME: wild hydrangea, seven barks, common hydrangea, *Hydrangea vulgaris.*
OCCURRENCE: native to the United States and is cultivated across the world as a garden plant.
PARTS USED: the root which contains two resins, gum, sugar,

starch, sulphuric and phosphoric acids and a glucoside called hydrangin.

MEDICINAL USES: diuretic, cathartic, tonic, nephritic. This herb is very good at preventing and removing stones in the urinary system, and relieving the pain due to urinary gravel. The fluid extract is also used to correct alkaline urine, chronic vaginal discharges and irritation of the bladder in older people. This drug was used by native American Indians and its benefits were passed on to European settlers.

ADMINISTERED AS: fluid extract, decoction, syrup.

Iceland moss *Cetraria islandica.*

COMMON NAME: Iceland lichen, cetraria.

OCCURRENCE: indigenous to a wide area of the northern hemisphere.

PARTS USED: the dried whole lichen. The moss contains a large quantity of starchy mater called lichenin as well as fumaric acid,oxalic acid and iodine.

MEDICINAL USES: demulcent, tonic, nutritive. The lichen has antibiotic properties and used to be given for tuberculosis as it was reputed to kill the tubercle bacillus, and clear phlegm from the lungs. It is used today for asthma, other respiratory problems and to soothe the digestive tract, stopping nausea. It is also used as a food, once the bitter principles are removed by boiling.

ADMINISTERED AS: decoction, dietary item.

Ipecacuanha *Cephaelis ipecacuanha.*

COMMON NAME: *Psychotria ipecacuanha.*

OCCURRENCE: native to Brazil, Bolivia and parts of South America and was introduced into Europe in the seventeenth century.

PARTS USED: the chief constituents of the root are the alkaloids emetrine, cephaelin and psychotrine, as well as two glucosides, choline, resin, calcium oxalate and a volatile oil among other compounds.

MEDICINAL USES: diaphoretic, emetic, expectorant, stimulant. The effects of the drug on the body are entirely dependent on the dose given. In very small doses, ipecacuanha stimulates the stomach, liver and intestine aiding digestion and increasing appetite while in slightly larger doses it has diaphoretic and expectorant properties which is good for colds, coughs and dysentery. Large doses of the drug are emetic. There is a lot of historical use of this drug against amoebic (or tropical) dysentery where rapid cures can occur. Care should be taken in utilizing this drug as emetine can have a toxic effect on the heart, blood vessels, lungs and intestines and cause severe illness.

ADMINISTERED AS: powdered root, fluid extract, tincture, syrup.

Irish moss *Chondrus crispus.*

COMMON NAME: carrageen, chondrus, carrahan, carragheen.

OCCURRENCE: common at low tide on all shores of the North Atlantic.

PARTS USED: the dried plant which contains mucilage and sulphur compounds.

MEDICINAL USES: demulcent, pectoral, emollient; nutritive. A popular remedy which is made into a jelly for pulmonary complaints, kidney and bladder diseases. It is widely used as a culinary article.

ADMINISTERED AS: dietary item.

Ivy *Hedera helix.*

COMMON NAME: common ivy.

OCCURRENCE: native to many parts of Europe and northern and central Asia.

PARTS USED: the leaves and berries.

MEDICINAL USES: stimulating, diaphoretic, cathartic. The leaves have been used as poultices on enlarged glands, ulcers and abscesses and the berries ease fevers and were used extensively during the Great Plague of London.
ADMINISTERED AS: poultice, infusion.

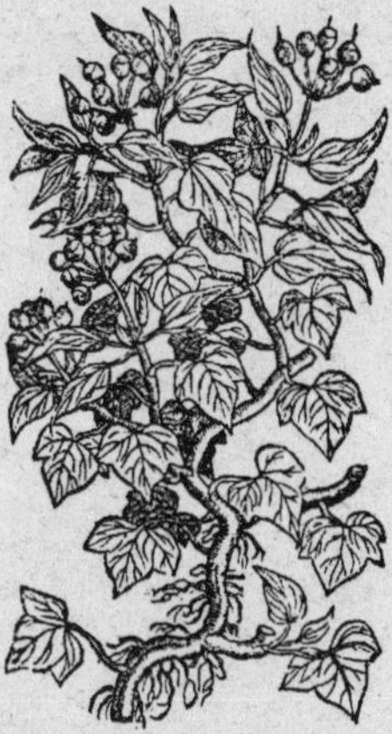

common ivy

Ivy, Ground *Glechoma hederacea.*
COMMON NAME: alehoof, gill-go-over-the-ground, haymaids, tun-hoof, hedgemaids, coltsfoot, robin-run-in-the-hedge.
OCCURRENCE: very common on hedges and waste ground all over Britain.
PARTS USED: the whole herb.
MEDICINAL USES: diuretic, astringent, tonic and gently stimulant. It is good in relieving kidney diseases and indigestion. Ground ivy tea is useful in pectoral complaints and in weakness of the digestive organs. The expressed juice, when sniffed up the nose, is said to successfully cure a headache and can be administered externally to ease bruises and black eyes. It also has antiscorbutic qualities.
ADMINISTERED AS: fluid extract, expressed juice and infusion.

Ivy, Poison *Rhus toxicodendron.*
COMMON NAME: poison oak, poison vine.
OCCURRENCE: native to the United States of America.
PARTS USED: the fresh leaves which contain a resin called toxicodendron as the active principle.
MEDICINAL USES: irritant, rubefacient, stimulant, narcotic. This herb

is successful in treating obstinate skin eruptions, palsy, paralysis, acute rheumatism and joint stiffness. It has also been good in treating ringworm, allergic rashes and urinary incontinence. In small doses, poison ivy is a very good sedative for the nervous system, but care must be taken in its use as it can trigger gastric and intestinal irritation, drowsiness, stupor and delirium.
Administered as: tincture, fluid extract, infusion.

Jaborandi *Pilocarpus microphyllus.*
Common name: arruda do mato, arruda brava, jamguarandi, juarandi.
Occurrence: a native Brazilian plant.
Parts used: the dried leaves. The main constituents of the leaves are a volatile oil and three alkaloids—pilocarpine, isopilocarpine, pilocarpidine.
Medicinal uses: stimulant, diaphoretic, expectorant. This herb is used as the crude drug and as the purified alkaloid, pilocarpine. Jaborandi is used for psoriasis, deafness, baldness, chronic catarrh, tonsillitis, dropsy and catarrhal jaundice. It can also benefit fat removal from the heart in heart disease, pleurisy, chronic renal diseases and reducing thirst in fevered patients. The extracted alkaloid, Pilocarpine, has an antagonistic effect to atropine, from belladonna, *Atropa belladonna* and other related plants, and causes contraction of the pupil of the eye. It is used as a fast and highly effective diaphoretic drug, increasing gland secretions and the flow of breast milk. Both the jaborandi and pilocarpine can irritate the stomach, causing vomiting even when given as an injection, so care should be advised upon using this drug.
Administered as: powdered leaves, tincture, injection, fluid extract.

Jacob's ladder *Polemonicum coeruleum.*
Common name: Greek valerian, charity.

OCCURRENCE: found wild in ditches and streams across England and southern Scotland.
PARTS USED: the herb.
MEDICINAL USES: diaphoretic, astringent, alterative, expectorant. A useful drug in fevers and inflammatory diseases, pleurisy, etc. It induces copious perspiration and eases coughs, colds, bronchial and lung complaints.
ADMINISTERED AS: an infusion.

Jewelweed *Impatiens aurea, Impatiens biflora.*
COMMON NAME: wild balsam, balsamweed, pale-touch-me-not, slipperweed, silverweed, wild lady's slipper, speckled jewels, wild celandine, quick in the hand, *Impatiens pallida, I. fulva.*
OCCURRENCE: members of the genus *Impatiens* are found distributed across the northern temperate zone and South Africa; mostly natives of mountainous regions in tropical Asia and Africa.
PARTS USED: the herb.
MEDICINAL USES: aperient, diuretic, emetic, cathartic. The diuretic qualities of the herb make it useful against dropsy and jaundice while the fresh juice is reputed to remove warts, corns and cure ringworm. The fresh herb was made into an ointment with lard and used for piles. Due to its acrid taste and strong action, jewelweed is rarely used in herbal medicine today.
ADMINISTERED AS: expressed juice, ointment.

Juniper *Juniperus communis.*
OCCURRENCE: a common shrub native to Great Britain and widely distributed through many parts of the world.
PARTS USED: the berry and leaves.
MEDICINAL USES: the oil of juniper obtained from the ripe berries is stomachic, diuretic and carminative and is used to treat indigestion, flatulence as well as kidney and bladder diseases. The main

use of juniper is in dropsy, and aiding other diuretic herbs to ease the disease.
ADMINISTERED AS: essential oil from berries, essential oil from wood, fluid extract, liquid extract, solid extract.

Kamala *Mallotus philippinensis.*
COMMON NAME: *Glandulae rottelerde*, kamcela, spoonwood, *Röttlera tinctoria*, kameela.
OCCURRENCE: native to India, Abyssinia, southern Arabia, China and Australia.
PARTS USED: the powder removed from the capsular fruit, composed of hairs and glands.
MEDICINAL USES: taeniafuge, purgative. The powder kills and expels tapeworms from the body. The worm is usually removed whole. It is a quick and active purgative drug, causing griping and nausea. It is used externally for cutaneous complaints including scabies and herpetic ringworm.
ADMINISTERED AS: powdered kamala, fluid extract.

Kava-kava *Piper methysticum.*
COMMON NAME: ava, ava pepper, kava, intoxicating pepper.
OCCURRENCE: indigenous to Polynesia, Sandwich Islands, South Sea Islands and Australian colonies.
PARTS USED: the peeled, dried rhizome. The plant contains two resins, one called kavine, a volatile oil, starch and an alkaloid termed kavaine methysticcum yangonin.
MEDICINAL USES: tonic, stimulant, diuretic. There is a long history of use against gonorrhoea, vaginitis, leucorrhoea, nocturnal incontinence and other problems of the urinary-genital tract. As a strong diuretic, kava is good for gout, rheumatism, bronchial problems and heart trouble. Kava acts on the nerve centres in a stimulating, then depressing manner, and has been used as a local anaesthetic as it

causes paralysis of the respiratory centre. It relieves pain and has an aphrodisiac effect.
ADMINISTERED AS: powdered root, fluid extract, solid extract.

Knapweed, Greater *Centaurea scabiosa.*
COMMON NAME: hardhead, ironhead, hard irons, churls head, logger head, horse knops, mat fellon, bottleweed, bullweed, cowede, bottsede.
OCCURRENCE: a perennial plant frequently seen in field borders and waste ground in England, but rare in Scotland.
PARTS USED: the root and seeds.
MEDICINAL USES: diuretic, diaphoretic and tonic. Formerly greatly appreciated as a vulnerary herb and used to cure loss of appetite. When taken as a decoction, it is good for catarrh; as an ointment for wounds, bruises and sores, etc.
ADMINISTERED AS: decoction and ointment.

Knotgrass *Polyganum ariculare.*
COMMON NAME: centuriode, ninety-knot, nine-joints, allseed, bird's tongue, sparrow tongue, red robin, armstrong, cowgrass, hogweed, pigrush, swynel grass, swine's grass.
OCCURRENCE: native around the globe; abundant on arable land, waste ground and roadside verges.
PARTS USED: the whole herb.
MEDICINAL USES: astringent, diuretic, anthelmintic, vulnerary and styptic. An infusion of the herb was used in diarrhoea, bleeding haemorrhoids and all haemorrhages. As a diuretic, it was said to expel stones and also parasitic worms. The fresh juice stops nosebleeds, if squirted up the nose and applied to the temples. As an ointment, it heals sores very well.
ADMINISTERED AS: expressed juice, infusion, decoction and ointment.

Kola nuts *Kola vera.*

COMMON NAME: guru nut, cola, kola seeds, gurru nuts, bissy nuts, cola seeds, *Cola acuminata*, *Sterculia acuminata.*

OCCURRENCE: native to Sierra Leone and North Ashanti and cultivated in tropical western Africa, West Indies, Brazil and Java.

PARTS USED: the seeds.

MEDICINAL USES: nerve stimulant, diuretic, cardiac tonic. This drug is a good overall tonic, largely due to the caffeine it contains. It has been used as a remedy for diarrhoea and for those with an alcoholic habit.

ADMINISTERED AS: powdered seeds, tincture, fluid and solid extract.

Laburnum *Cytisus laburnam.*

COMMON NAME: yellow laburnum.

OCCURRENCE: indigenous to high mountain regions of Europe and widely cultivated across the globe as a garden plant.

PARTS USED: the alkaloid, obtained from the plant, called cytisine.

MEDICINAL USES: all parts of the laburnum are thought to be poisonous, particularly the seeds. The alkaloid has been recommended in whooping cough and asthma, and also as an insecticide, but it has not been used due to the very poisonous nature of the compound. Laburnum poisoning symptoms include intense sleepiness, vomiting, convulsive movements, coma and unequally dilated pupils. Laburnum is also poisonous to cattle and horses and deaths of both livestock and humans have resulted from ingestion of this plant.

Lady's mantle *Alchemilla vulgaris.*

COMMON NAME: lion's foot, bear's foot, nine hooks, stellaria.

OCCURRENCE: native to mountainous districts of Britain and widely distributed over northern or Arctic Europe, Asia and Greenland.

PARTS USED: the herb.
MEDICINAL USES: astringent, styptic, vulnerary. Herbalists used to say that lady's mantle was one of the best herbs for wounds. In modern times, it is used as a cure for excessive menstruation as an infusion or injection. The root is very good for stopping all bleeding and may also act as a violent purge. The herb is also said to promote quiet sleep.
ADMINISTERED AS: decoction, infusion, injection, tincture, fluid extract, dried root.

Larch *Pinus larix.*
COMMON NAME: *Larix europaea*, *Abies larix*, *Larix decidua*, *Laricus cortex*, European larch, Venice turpentine.
OCCURRENCE: indigenous to hilly regions of central Europe, but was introduced into Britain in 1639.
PARTS USED: the inner bark which contains tannic acid, larixinic acid and turpentine.
MEDICINAL USES: stimulant, diuretic, astringent, balsamic and expectorant. It is very useful as an external application for eczema and psoriasis. However, it is mainly used as a stimulant expectorant in chronic bronchitis, internal haemorrhage and cystitis. Larch turpentine has also been suggested as an antidote in cyanide or opium poisoning and has been used as a hospital disinfectant.
ADMINISTERED AS: fluid extract or syrup.

Larkspur *Delphinicum consolida.*
COMMON NAME: field larkspur, lark's chaw, lark's heel, knight's spur, lark's toe.
OCCURRENCE: found wild in fields through Europe and Great Britain.
PARTS USED: the seeds. The active principle in the plant is delphinine, an irritant poison also found in STAVESACRE.

MEDICINAL USES: parasiticide, insecticide. The tincture of the seeds is used to destroy lice and nits in the hair and given internally in spasmodic asthma and dropsy. The expressed juice from the leaves was applied to bleeding piles and an infusion of the whole plant was said to benefit colic.
ADMINISTERED AS: infusion, tincture, expressed juice.

Laurel *Laurus nobilis*.
COMMON NAME: bay, sweet bay, true laurel, laurier d'apollon, roman laurel, noble laurel, lorbeer, laurier sauce, daphne.
OCCURRENCE: native to the shores of the Mediterranean and cultivated in Britain.
PARTS USED: the leaves, fruit and essential oil. The volatile oil contains pinene, geraniol, eugenol, cineol, bitter principles and tannin.
MEDICINAL USES: stomachic, narcotic, diaphoretic, emetic. In ancient times, laurel was highly valued as a medicine but now laurel is only selectively utilized. The leaves were formerly used in hysteria, flatulent colic and in treating the absence of menstrual periods, but now are only used to stimulate the digestion. The oil of bays is also used for earache, sprains and bruises and rheumatism.
ADMINISTERED AS: essential oil, infusion.

Lavender, English *Lavandula vera*.
OCCURRENCE: indigenous to mountainous regions in the western Mediterranean and is cultivated extensively in France, Italy, England and Norway.
PARTS USED: the flowers and the essential oil which contains linalool, linalyl acetate, cineol, pinene, limonene and tannin.
MEDICINAL USES: aromatic, carminative, stimulant, nervine. It is mainly used as a flavouring agent for disagreeable odours in oint-

ments or syrups. The essential oil when taken internally is restorative and a tonic against faintness, heart palpitations, giddiness and colic. It raises the spirits, promotes the appetite and dispels flatulence. When applied externally, the oil relieves toothache, neuralgia, sprains and rheumatism. The oil is utilized widely in aromatherapy, often to very beneficial effects.
ADMINISTERED AS: fluid extract, tincture, essential oil, spirit, infusion, tea, poultice, distilled water.

Lemon *Citrus limonica.*
COMMON NAME: limon, *Citrus medica*, *Citrus Limonum*, citronnier, neemoo, leemoo, limoun, limone.
OCCURRENCE: indigenous to northern India and widely cultivated in Mediterranean countries.
PARTS USED: the fruit, rind, juice and oil. Lemon peel contains an essential oil and a bitter principle, while lemon juice is rich in citric acid, sugar and gum. Oil of lemon contains the aldehyde, citral and the oils pinene and citronella.
MEDICINAL USES: antiscorbutic, tonic, refrigerant, cooling. Lemon juice is the best preventative drug for scurvy and is also very valuable in fevers and allaying thirst. It is recommended in acute rheumatism and may be given to counteract narcotic poisons such as opium. It is used as an astringent gargle in sore throats, for uterine haemorrhage after childbirth, as a lotion in sunburn and as a cure for severe hiccoughs. The juice is also good for jaundice and heart palpitations. A decoction of lemon is a good antiperiodic drug and can be used to replace quinine in malarial injections, or to reduce the temperature in typhoid fever. Lemon oil is a strong external rubefacient and also has stomachic and carminative qualities.
ADMINISTERED AS: syrup, decoction, fresh juice, tincture, essential oil, dietary item.

Lettuce, Wild *Lactuca virosa.*
COMMON NAME: lachicarium, strong-scented lettuce, green endive, lettuce opium, acrid lettuce, laitue vireuse.
OCCURRENCE: found in western and southern Europe, including Great Britain.
PARTS USED: the leaves, dried milk juice—lactuarium. Lactuarium is obtained by cutting the stem in sections and collecting the latex juice. It turns reddish-brown in colour when dried.
MEDICINAL USES: anodyne, sedative, narcotic, mild diaphoretic, diuretic. The drug resembles a weak opium, without opium's tendency to upset the digestive system. It is used to allay irritable coughs and as a sedative and narcotic, but only infrequently. It is also used for dropsy, inducing sleep and easing colic.
ADMINISTERED AS: powder, tincture, fluid extract, syrup, alcoholic extract.

Lilac *Syringa vulgaris.*
COMMON NAME: common lilac.
OCCURRENCE: a shrub native to Persia and the mountains of eastern Europe.
PARTS USED: the leaves and fruit.
MEDICINAL USES: as a vermifuge, tonic, antiperiodic and febrifuge. It may be used as a substitute for ALOES (*Aloe vera/Aloe perryi*) and in the treatment of malaria.
ADMINISTERED AS: an infusion.

Lily of the valley *Convallaria magalis.*
COMMON NAME: May lily, convarraria, Our Lady's tears, convallily, lily constancy, ladder to heaven, Jacob's ladder.
OCCURRENCE: native to Europe and distributed over North America and northern Asia. A very localized plant in England and Scotland.
PARTS USED: the flowers, leaves and whole herb. The chief con-

stituents are two glucosides—convallamarin (the active principle) and convallarin, as well as tannin and mineral salts.

MEDICINAL USES: cardiac tonic, diuretic. A similar drug to digitalis, from the FOXGLOVE, although it is less powerful. Strongly recommended in valvular heart disease, cardiac debility, dropsy and it slows the action of a weak, irritated heart. Lily of the valley does not have accumulatory effects and can be taken in full and frequent doses without harm. A decoction of the flowers is good at removing obstructions in the urinary canal.

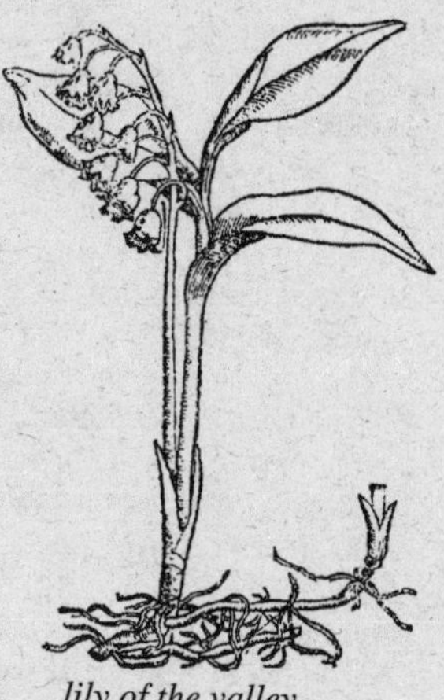

lily of the valley

ADMINISTERED AS: fluid extracts, decoction tincture, powdered flowers.

Lily, Madonna *Lilium candidum.*

COMMON NAME: white lily, meadow lily.

OCCURRENCE: a southern European native which has been cultivated in Great Britain and America for centuries.

PARTS USED: the bulb.

MEDICINAL USES: demulcent, astringent, mucilaginous. The bulb is mainly used as an emollient poultice for ulcers, tumours and external inflammation. When made into an ointment, Madonna lily removes corns and eliminates pain and inflammation from burns and scalds, reducing scarring. When used in combination with life root (*Senecio aureus*), Madonnna lily is of great value

in treating leucorrhoea, prolapse of the womb and other female complaints. The bulb is eaten as food in Japan.
ADMINISTERED AS: poultice, ointment, decoction.

Lime fruit *Citrus medica* var. *acida*.
COMMON NAME: *Citrus acris*, *Citrus acida*, limettae fructus.
OCCURRENCE: a native Asian tree which is cultivated in many warm countries including the West Indies and Italy.
PARTS USED: the fruit and juice.
MEDICINAL USES: refrigerant, antiscorbutic. The juice of the lime contains citric acid and is a popular beverage, sweetened as a syrup. It is used to treat dyspepsia.
ADMINISTERED AS: fresh juice, syrup.

Lime tree *Tilia europoea*.
COMMON NAME: linden flowers, linn flowers, common lime, tilleul, flores tiliae, *Tilia vulgaris*, *T. intermedia*, *T. cordata*, *T. platyphylla*.
OCCURRENCE: native to the British Isles and the northern temperate zone.
PARTS USED: the lime flowers, bark, powdered charcoal. The flowers contain volatile oil, flavonid glucosides, saponins, condensed tannins and mucilage.
MEDICINAL USES: nervine, stimulant, tonic. An infusion of the flowers is good for indigestion, hysteria, nervous vomiting, colds, 'flu and catarrh. They can also help calm overactive children and relax the nervous system. Lime flower tea eases headaches and insomnia. The flowers are said to lower blood pressure (possibly due to the bioflavonids they contain) and are said to remedy arteriosclerosis. The inner bark of the lime has a diuretic effect and is utilized for gout and kidney stones as well as treating coronary artery disease by dilating the coronary arteries. The powdered

charcoal was used in gastric and dyspeptic disorders and applied to burnt or sore areas.

ADMINISTERED AS: infusion, powdered charcoal, dried inner bark, tea.

Liquorice *Glycyrrhiza glabra.*

COMMON NAME: licorice, lycorys, *Liquiriha officinalis.*

OCCURRENCE: a shrub native to south-east Europe and south-west Asia and cultivated in the British Isles.

PARTS USED: the root. The chief compound in the root is glychrrhizin along with sugar, starch, gum, asparagus, tannin and resin.

MEDICINAL USES: demulcent, pectoral, emollient. A very popular and well-known remedy for coughs, consumption and chest complaints. Liquorice extract is included in cough lozenges and pastilles, with sedatives and expectorants. An infusion of bruised root and FLAX (linseed) is good for irritable coughs, sore throats and laryngitis. Liquorice is used to a greater extent as a medicine in China and other eastern countries. The herb is used by brewers to give colour to porter and stout and is employed in the manufacture of chewing or smoking tobacco.

ADMINISTERED AS: powdered root, fluid extract, infusion, solid extract.

Liverwort, English *Peltigera canina.*

COMMON NAME: lichen caninus, lichen cinereus terrestris, ash-coloured ground liverwort, liverleaf, *Hepatica triloba.*

OCCURRENCE: grows in moist, shady places in Britain and Europe.

PARTS USED: the whole lichen.

MEDICINAL USES: deobstruent, slightly purgative, *Peltigera canina* is held in esteem as a cure for liver complaints and was formerly regarded as a remedy for hydrophobia.

ADMINISTERED AS: infusion and fluid extract.

Lobelia *Lobelia inflata.*
COMMON NAME: Indian tobacco, asthma weed, pukeweed, jagroot, vomitwort, bladderpod, *Rapuntium inflatum.*
OCCURRENCE: native to North America and grown in British gardens for many years.
PARTS USED: the herb, which contains the alkaloids, lobeline, isolobeline, lobelanidine and lobinaline along with fixed oil, gum, resin and lignin.
MEDICINAL USES: expectorant, emetic, diaphoretic, anti-asthmatic, stimulant. The use of this plant was passed to Europeans from native American Indians and it has been used as a major relaxant remedy used to treat pain caused by muscle spasms. Thus it is highly effective against asthma, bronchial complaints and lung problems. Lobelia may be given to ease convulsive and inflammatory disorders such as epilepsy, tonsillitis, diphtheria and tetanus. Externally, the herb is used for eye complaints, insect bites, POISON IVY irritation, ringworm, sprains, bruises and muscle spasms. The use of lobelia as an emetic is debatable as to whether it would benefit the patient, and its use is encouraged or discouraged by different herbals. Lobelia is a very important herbal remedy in modern usage.
ADMINISTERED AS: tincture, infusion, powdered bark, syrup and fluid extract.

Loosestrife *Lysimachia vulgaris.*
COMMON NAME: yellow loosestrife, yellow willow herb, herb willow, willow-wort, wood pimpernel.
OCCURRENCE: grows in shady banks and riversides in England.
PARTS USED: the herb.
MEDICINAL USES: astringent, expectorant. This herb is good at stopping bleeding of any kind, particularly of the mouth, nose and wounds. It is also used to restrain profuse menstrual bleeding and

calm severe diarrhoea. Distilled water made with loosestrife was utilized to clean ulcers and reduce inflammation and to clear spots, marks and scabs from the skin. An infusion was used as a gargle in relaxed throat and quinsy.
ADMINISTERED AS: distilled water, dried herb, infusion and ointment.

Lovage *Levisticum officinale.*
COMMON NAME: *Ligusticum levisticum*, old English lovage, Italian lovage, Cornish lovage, Chinese tang kui, man-mu.
OCCURRENCE: one of the old English herbs which was very generally cultivated; it was not indigenous to Great Britain but native to the Mediterranean region.
PARTS USED: the root, leaves, young stems and seeds. The plant contains a volatile oil, angelic acid, a bitter extract and resin.
MEDICINAL USES: the young stems are used in a similar manner to ANGELICA for flavouring and confectionery. The roots and fruits are aromatic, stimulant, diuretic and carminative in action. They are generally used in stomach disorders, and feverish attacks including those with colic and flatulence. The fresh leaves are eaten as a salad and when dried are infused into a pleasant tea with emmenagogue properties. An infusion of the root was recommended by old herbalists for gravel, jaundice and urinary problems and the sudorific nature of the roots and seeds meant they were highly favoured in treating "pestilential disorders".
ADMINISTERED AS: infusion of leaves and root infusion.

Lucerne *Medicago sativa.*
COMMON NAME: purple medick, cultivated lucern, alfalfa, purple medicle.
OCCURRENCE: an ancient herb, of unknown origin. Cultivated in Europe, Great Britain, Peru and Persia for hundreds of years.

Parts used: the herb.
Medicinal uses: this herb is used, as an infusion, to encourage weight gain and flesh development. It has also been used to feed cattle and horses.
Administered as: infusion.

Lungwort *Sticta pulmonaria.*
Common name: Jerusalem cowslip, oak lungs, lung moss.
Occurrence: found in Europe, but uncommon in woods in Britain.
Parts used: the whole lichen.
Medicinal uses: astringent, mucilaginous, pectoral, healing. It is very valuable in treating coughs, lung complaints and asthma. It is also good at reducing inflammation and pain.
Administered as: liquid extract, infusion.

Lupin, White *Lupinus albus.*
Common name: lupine, wolfsbohne.
Occurrence: native to southern Europe and parts of Asia and is now extensively cultivated in Italy.
Parts used: the seeds, herb. The main compounds within the plant are the glucoside, lupinin; the alkaloids lupinidine and luparine.
Medicinal uses: anthelmintic, diuretic, emmenagogue. The bruised seeds, when soaked in water, are applied to ulcers and sores and when taken internally the seeds kill parasitic worms and excite the menstrual discharge. It was used by the Romans as food and can also be used for fibres to make cloth, paper and adhesive.
Administered as: poultice, infusion.

Mace *Myristica fragrans.*
Common name: macis, muscadier, *Arillus myristicae*, *Myristica officinalis*, *Myristica moschata.*

OCCURRENCE: native to the Molucca Islands, New Guinea, Bondy Islands and introduced into Sri Lanka and the West Indies.
PARTS USED: the growth outside the shell of the nutmeg seed—called the arillus. The main constituents of mace are a volatile oil, protein, gum, resins, sugars and two fixed oils. The volatile oil contains a lot of pinene and some myristicin.
MEDICINAL USES: stimulant, tonic, carminative, flavouring agent. This herb is used to help digestion and stomach weakness and increase the blood circulation and body temperature. Mace has been used against putrid and pestilential fevers and, combined with other herbs, intermittent fevers.
ADMINISTERED AS: powdered herb.

Magnolia *Magnolia Virginiana.*
COMMON NAME: cucumber tree, blue magnolia, swamp sassfras, *Magnolia glauca, M. acuminata, M. tripetata.*
OCCURRENCE: native to the USA but is cultivated in Great Britain.
PARTS USED: the bark of stem and root.
MEDICINAL USES: mild, diaphoretic, tonic, aromatic, stimulant. The bark is used against rheumatism and malaria, and the cones of the tree are steeped in spirit to make a tonic tincture. A warm infusion of bark is laxative and sudorific while a cold infusion is antiperiodic and tonic in effect.
ADMINISTERED AS: tincture, infusion, fluid extract.

Maidenhair *Adiantum capillus-veneris.*
COMMON NAME: true maidenhair, hair of Venus, rock fern, capillaire common or capillaire de Montpellier.
OCCURRENCE: this grows wild in southern Europe and southern and central Britain.
PARTS USED: the herb, which contains tannin and mucilage but has not yet been fully investigated.

MEDICINAL USES: pectoral, expectorant, mucilaginous. The fern has been used as a remedy in chest complaints, coughs and throat problems. It is an ingredient of cough mixtures, its flavour masked by sugar and ORANGE-FLOWER water. Maidenhair is good at easing pulmonary catarrh and is used in Europe as an emmenagogue.
ADMINISTERED AS: infusion, syrup.

Male fern *Dryopteris felix-mas.*
COMMON NAME: *Aspidium felix-mas*, male shield fern.
OCCURRENCE: grows in all areas of Europe, temperate Asia, North India, North and South Africa, the temperate areas of the United States and the South American Andes.
PARTS USED: the root and the oil extracted from it. The oil is extracted using ether and contains the acid, filmaron, filicic acid, tannin, resin and sugar.
MEDICINAL USES: anthelmintic, vermifuge, taeniafuge. It is probably the best drug against tapeworm, it is normally given at night after several hours of fasting. When followed by a purgative drug in the morning, e.g. CASTOR OIL very good results are obtained. The size of the dose administered must be carefully assessed as male fern is an irritant poison in too large a dose, causing muscle weakness, coma and possible damage to the eyesight.
ADMINISTERED AS: powdered root, fluid extract; oil of male fern.

Mandrake *Atropa mandragora.*
COMMON NAME: mandragora, Satan's apple.
OCCURRENCE: a plant native to southern Europe but it can be cultivated in Great Britain.
PARTS USED: the herb and root.
MEDICINAL USES: emetic, purgative, cooling, anodyne, hypnotic. The fresh root is a very powerful emetic and purgative drug and

the dried bark of the root also shares the purgative qualities. Ancient herbalists used mandrake to kill pain and to give rest and sleep to patients, as well as using it for melancholy, convulsions, rheumatic pain and scrofulous tumours. They administered the drug as the bark of the root, expressed juice or as an infusion of the root. In large doses, mandrake was said to cause delirium and madness. The herb was used as an anaesthetic in ancient Greek medicine.
ADMINISTERED AS: infusion, fresh root, powdered bark, expressed juice.

Maple, Red *Acer rubrum.*
COMMON NAME: swamp maple, curled maple.
OCCURRENCE: a native American tree, introduced into Britain in 1656 as an ornamental tree.
PARTS USED: the bark.
MEDICINAL USES: astringent. The native American Indians used an infusion of the bark as an application for sore eyes.
ADMINISTERED AS: an infusion.

Mare's tail *Hippuris vulgaris.*
COMMON NAME: female horsetail, marsh barren horsetail.
OCCURRENCE: a native British aquatic flowering plant found in shallow ponds, rivers, ditches and lake margins.
PARTS USED: the herb.
MEDICINAL USES: vulnerary. Old herbalists viewed mare's tail as good for stopping bleeding, be it internal or external. It was said to be used to heal ulcers, green wounds in children, ruptures and urinary stones. The herb was also used to strengthen the intestinal system, for head colds and as a warm poultice on skin eruptions and inflammations.
ADMINISTERED AS: poultice, decoction.

Marigold *Calendula officinalis.*
COMMON NAME: *Caltha officinalis*, golds, ruddes, marg gowles, oculus Christi, marygold, garden marigold, solis sponsa.
OCCURRENCE: a native of southern Europe and a common garden plant in Great Britain.
PARTS USED: the petals and herb. Only the deep orange-flowered variety is of medicinal use.
MEDICINAL USES: stimulant, diaphoretic. Mainly used as a local remedy. Taken internally, an infusion of the herb prevents pus formation and externally is good in cleaning chronic ulcers and varicose veins. Formerly considered to be of benefit as an aperient and detergent to clear visceral obstructions and jaundice. A marigold flower, when rubbed onto a bee or wasp sting, was known to relieve pain and reduce swelling, while a lotion from the flowers was good for inflamed and sore eyes. The expressed juice of the plant was used to clear headaches and remove warts.
ADMINISTERED AS: infusion, distilled water and lotion.

Marjoram *Origanum vulgare*
OCCURRENCE: generally distributed over Asia, Europe and North Africa and also found freely in England.
PARTS USED: the herb and volatile oil.
MEDICINAL USES: the oil has stimulant, carminative, diaphoretic, mildly tonic and emmenagogue qualities. As a warm infusion, it is used to produce perspiration and bring out the spots of measles as well as giving relief from spasms, colic and dyspeptic pain. The oil has been used externally as a rubefacient and liniment, and on cotton wool placed next to an aching tooth it relieves the pain. The dried herb may be utilized as a hot poultice for swellings, rheumatism and colic, while an infusion of the fresh plant will ease a nervous headache.
ADMINISTERED AS: essential oil, poultice and infusion.

Marjoram, Sweet *Origanum marjorana.*
COMMON NAME: knotted marjoram, *Majorana hortensis.*
OCCURRENCE: native to Portugal and grown as an annual plant through the rest of Europe and Great Britain.
PARTS USED: the herb and leaves. The plant contains tannic acid, mucilage, bitter substances and an essential oil.
MEDICINAL USES: tonic, stimulant, emmenagogue. The essential oil, oleum majoranae when extracted from the leaves, makes a good external application for sprains and bruises, and acts as an emmenagogue when taken internally. Sweet marjoram is widely used in cookery and aids digestion of food.
ADMINISTERED AS: essential oil, dried or fresh leaves.

Marshmallow *Althaea officinalis.*
COMMON NAME: mallards, mauls, schloss tea, cheeses, mortification, root, guimauve.
OCCURRENCE: a native of Europe, found in salt marshes, meadows, ditches and riverbanks. It is locally distributed in England and has been introduced to Scotland.
PARTS USED: the leaves, root and flowers. Marshmallow contains starch, mucilage, pectin, oil, sugar, asparagin, glutinous matter and cellulose.
MEDICINAL USES: demulcent, emollient. Very useful in inflammation and irritation of the alimentary canal and the urinary and respiratory organs. A decoction of the root is effective against sprains, bruises of any muscle aches. When boiled in milk or wine marshmallow relieves diseases of the chest, e.g. coughs, bronchitis or whooping cough and it eases the bowels after dysentery without any astringent effects. It is frequently given as a syrup to infants and children.
ADMINISTERED AS: infusion, decoction, syrup, fluid extract.

Masterwort *Imperatoria ostruthium.*
OCCURRENCE: native to central Europe and alpine regions; cultivated in Great Britain for many years.
PARTS USED: the rhizome.
MEDICINAL USES: stimulant, antispasmodic, carminative. Masterwort has been used in asthma, stroke, dyspepsia and menstrual problems. A decoction of the herb in urine was considered beneficial against dropsy, cramp, epilepsy, flatulence, gout and kidney and uterine problems.
ADMINISTERED AS: distilled water, decoction, fluid extract.

Mastic *Pistacia lentiscus.*
COMMON NAME: mastich, lentisk.
OCCURRENCE: indigenous to the Mediterranean regions of Spain, Portugal, France, Greece, Turkey, tropical Africa and the Canary Islands.
PARTS USED: the resin, which contains a volatile oil, an alcohol-insoluble resin and an alcohol-soluble resin.
MEDICINAL USES: stimulant, diuretic. Similar to TURPENTINE in effect, but its use in medicine has declined. In some areas it is used for diarrhoea in children, or chewed to sweeten the breath. Today, mastic is mainly used as a filling for carious teeth.
ADMINISTERED AS: resin.

Matico *Piper angustifolium.*
COMMON NAME: soldier's herb, thoho-thoho, moho-moho, *Artanthe elongata*, *Stephensia elongata*, *Piper granulosium*, matica.
OCCURRENCE: native to Peru and spread over much of tropical America. It has been grown in England.
PARTS USED: the dried leaves which contain a volatile oil, artanthic acid, tannin and resin.
MEDICINAL USES: astringent, stimulant, styptic, diuretic. It is rec-

ommended for chronic mucous discharges, leucorrhoea, haemorrhoids, diarrhoea, dysentery and urinary and genital complaints. The leaves stop bleeding from most sites, and are used as an application to slight wounds, ulcers, bites from leeches or after teeth extraction.
ADMINISTERED AS: dried leaves, fluid extract.

Mayweed *Anthemis cotula.*
COMMON NAME: maroute, cotula, dog chamomile, wild chamomile, foetid or stinking chamomile (or mayweed), dog's fennel, maithes, mathor, *Maruta cotula*, *Maruta foetida*, *Manzilla loca*, *Camomille puante*.
OCCURRENCE: frequently grows in fields and wild places in Great Britain and Europe.
PARTS USED: the flowers and leaves. The flowers contain volatile oil, oxalic, valeric and tannic acids, a bitter extractive and salts of iron, potassium, calcium and magnesium.
MEDICINAL USES: tonic, antispasmodic, emmenagogue and emetic. The smell of the flowers is still repulsive, but is less offensive than that of the rest of the plant, so the flowers are mainly used in medicine. It is used in hysteria, as a poultice for haemorrhoids and as an infusion in the bath. The flowers have also been used in sick headaches, menstrual problems, scrofula, gastric troubles and dy-sentery; to induce sleep in asthma and in convalescence after fevers.
ADMINISTERED AS: fluid extract, poultice, infusion, decoction.

Meadowsweet *Spiraea ulmaria.*
COMMON NAME: meadsweet, dolloff, queen of the meadow, bridewort, lady of the meadow.
OCCURRENCE: common in the British Isles in meadows or woods.
PARTS USED: the herb.
MEDICINAL USES: aromatic, astringent, diuretic, alterative. This herb

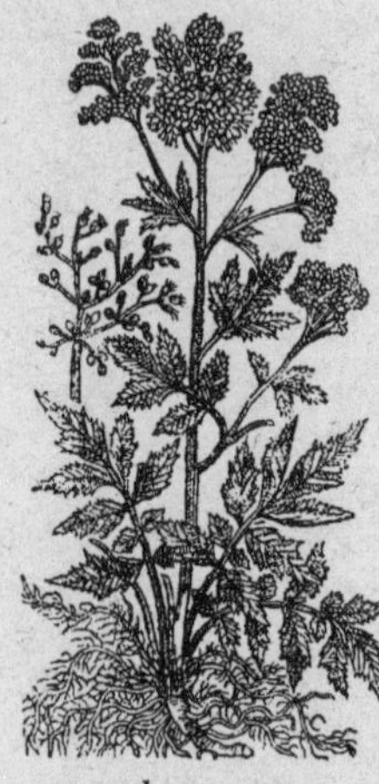
meadowsweet

is good against diarrhoea, stomach complaints and blood disorders. It is highly recommended for children's diarrhoea and dropsy and was used as a decoction ir wine to reduce fevers. Meadowsweet makes a pleasant everyday drink when infused and sweetened with honey. It is also included in many herb beers.
ADMINISTERED AS: infusion, decoction.

Melilot *Melilotus officinalis, Melilotus alba, Melilotus arvensis.*
COMMON NAME: king's clover, king's chafer, yellow melilot, white melilot, corn melilot, sweet clover, plaster clover, sweet lucerne, wild laburnham hart's tree.
OCCURRENCE: naturalized in all parts of the British Isles.
PARTS USED: the dried herb containing coumarin, hydrocoumaric acid, orthocoumaric acid and melilotic anhydride.
MEDICINAL USES: aromatic, emollient, carminative. When applied as a plaster, ointment or poultice, the herb is good at relieving abdominal or rheumatic pain. It is taken internally to relieve flatulence. The herb was formerly used for clearing the eyesight, headaches, wounds, ulcers and inflammation.
ADMINISTERED AS: poultice, expressed juice, infusion.

Mercury, Dog's *Mercurialis perennis.*
OCCURRENCE: a common plant in woods and shady places in Europe and Russian Asia.
PARTS USED: the herb.

MEDICINAL USES: purgative. Recommended for use externally to treat sore, watery eyes, deafness, pains in the ear, ague, jaundice and women's diseases. The fresh juice of the plant is used to remove warts and to cleanse inflammatory and discharging sores and swellings. A lotion is made for antiseptic external dressings while the juice is used as a nasal douche for catarrh.
ADMINISTERED AS: expressed juice, lotion, fresh herb.

Mescal buttons *Anhalonicum lewinii.*
COMMON NAME: *Lopophora lewinii*, *Analonium williamsii*, *Echinacactus lewinii*, *Echinocactus williamsii*, pellote, muscal buttons.
OCCURRENCE: Mexico and Texas.
PARTS USED: the tops of the cacti plant. The drug contains four alkaloids—anhalonine, mescaline, anhalonidine and lophophorine—as well as the chemicals pellotine and anhalamine.
MEDICINAL USES: cardiac, tonic, narcotic, emetic. The drug is useful in head injuries, hysteria, asthma, gout, neuralgia and rheumatism. The extracted compound pellotine has been used to induce sleep in people with insanity as it has no undesirable reactions. Large doses of mescal buttons produce an odd cerebral excitement, with visual disturbances. The physical effects include muscular relaxation, wakefulness, nausea, vomiting and dilation of the pupil. The ancient Aztec Indians believed mescal buttons to have divine properties and included its use to produce exaltation in their religious ceremonies.
ADMINISTERED AS: fluid extract, tincture, extracted alkaloid.

Mezereon *Daphne mezereum.*
COMMON NAME: spurge olive, spurge laurel, camolea, wolt schjeluke, kellernals, dwarf bay, flowering spurge, wild pepper, *Mezerei cortex*, *Mezerei officinarum*, *Laureole gentille*.

OCCURRENCE: indigenous to Britain, Europe and Siberia and was naturalized into the United States and Canada.
PARTS USED: the root, berries, the bark of the stem and root. The bark tastes acrid and this is due to a resin called mezeen. The other active chemicals are a fixed oil, a bitter glucoside called daphnin and a substance similar to euphorbone.
MEDICINAL USES: alterative, diuretic, stimulant, vesicant. An ointment of the bark is used to promote discharge from indolent ulcers, and it is also used for snake and other venomous bites. It is taken internally for chronic rheumatism, scrofula, syphilis, skin diseases and dropsy. The tincture is used to ease neuralgic pain and toothache. In large doses, it acts as an irritant poison and purgative drug causing vomiting, so care should be taken in monitoring the dose used.
ADMINISTERED AS: infusion, tincture, ointment.

Mistletoe *Viscum album.*
COMMON NAME: European mistletoe, bird lime mistletoe, herbe de la croix, mystyldene, lignum crucis.
OCCURRENCE: an evergreen, true parasitic plant found on several tree species including fruit and oak trees. It is found throughout Europe and Britain except in Scotland, where it is very rare.
PARTS USED: the leaves and young twigs. They contain mucilage, sugar, fixed oil, tannin and viscin, the active part of the plant.
MEDICINAL USES: nervine, antispasmodic, tonic and narcotic. It is highly recommended for epilepsy and other convulsive disorders, along with stopping internal haemorrhage. It has also been used in delirium, hysteria, neuralgia, nervous debility, urinary disorders and many other complaints arising from a weakened state of the nervous system. The berries are taken to cure severe stitches in the side, and the plant produces a sticky substance called bird-lime which is applied to ulcers and sores. Mistletoe is excellent for re-

ducing blood pressure and has been indicated to be a successful cure for chronic arthritis and in treating malignant tumours in the body.

ADMINISTERED AS: tincture, powdered leaves, infusion, fluid extract.

Motherwort *Leonurus cardiaca.*

COMMON NAME: lion's ear, lion's tail.

OCCURRENCE: a native plant in many parts of Europe, but only rarely found in the wild in Britain.

PARTS USED: the dried herb which contains the alkaloids leonurinine and stachydrine; the bitter glucosides leonurine and leonuridin, tannins and a volatile oil.

MEDICINAL USES: diaphoretic, antispasmodic, tonic, nervine, emmenagogue, sedative. An important use of the herb is in easing the anxiety after childbirth or at the menopause by lowering the blood pressure. It is excellent for female complaints by allaying nervous irritability, regulating menstruation and treating functional infertility. As a tonic, the herb acts well and is effective in treating fevers and allowing good recovery from them. Throughout history, Motherwort has been used to treat palpitations and rapid heart beat, particularly when they develop from anxiety or hysteria. As the name suggests, motherwort acts on the uterine system and the alkaloid stachydrine has the effect of hastening childbirth so this herb should not be used by pregnant women. It is beneficial, however, in causing the uterus to contract after delivery and in this manner is more effective than ERGOT.

ADMINISTERED AS: powdered herb, infusion, decoction, conserve.

Mountain flax *Linum catharticum.*

COMMON NAME: purging flax, dwarf flax, fairy flax, mill mountain.

OCCURRENCE: a common plant in meadows and pastures across Europe and Great Britain.

Parts used: the herb which contains a bitter resin and a crystalline principle called linin.
Medicinal uses: purgative, laxative, cathartic. It is a gentle cathartic drug with a laxative action preferred to senna. As an infusion, the dried herb has been used internally to treat muscular rheumatism and catarrhal infections. It can also be beneficial in liver complaints and jaundice.
Administered as: infusion, dried herb.

Mugwort *Artemisia vulgaris.*
Common name: felon herb, St. John's plant, moxa, cirigulum Sancti Johannis.
Occurrence: this grows wild in Great Britain on roadsides and hedgerows.
Parts used: the leaves, which contain volatile oil, flavonoids, tannin and a bitter principle called absinthin; the roots.
Medicinal uses: emmenagogue, stimulant, tonic, nervine, diuretic, diaphoretic. As a nervine, this herb is good in palsy, fits, epilepsy and for people with a feeble constitution. An infusion of the herb is used for intermittent fevers and the ague and given as a tonic. Mugwort's main use is as an emmenagogue to provoke delayed or absent periods and therefore it should not be used during pregnancy, except under the guidance of a qualified herbal practitioner. However, it does help during and after childbirth in speeding up the birth process and to expel the afterbirth. Mugwort acts on the digestive process and stimulates the liver and is used to treat gout and rheumatism. In China, the dried herb is burnt on or near the skin to stop rheumatic pain caused by damp and cold conditions. Also in China, mugwort is taken during pregnancy to prevent miscarriage, differing from the Western viewpoint.
Administered as: dried herb, fluid extract.

Mulberry *Monus nigra.*

COMMON NAME: common mulberry, black mulberry, purple mulberry.

OCCURRENCE: a native of Turkey, Armenia, Persia and is cultivated throughout Europe and Britain.

PARTS USED: the fruit which contains glucose, protein, pectin, tartaric and malic acids and ash.

MEDICINAL USES: laxative, refrigerant, nutritive. The fruit juice is a beneficial drink for convalescent people, as it checks the thirst and cools the blood after fevers. The fruits are made into wine, jam and conserve. The bark of the tree has a purgative and vermifuge effect on the body.

ADMINISTERED AS: syrup, expressed juice, infusion of bark.

Mullein *Verbascum thapsus.*

COMMON NAME: blanket herb, beggar's blanket, Aaron's rod, lady's foxglove, donkey's ears, torches, candlewick plant, wild ice leaf, Jupiter's staff, clown's lungwort, velvet plant, clot.

OCCURRENCE: widely distributed through Europe, temperate Asia, North America, Ireland and Great Britain.

PARTS USED: the leaves and flowers. The plant contains saponins, mucilage, gum volatile oil, flavonoids and glucosides.

MEDICINAL USES: demulcent, emollient, astringent, sedative, narcotic. This herb is very useful in pectoral

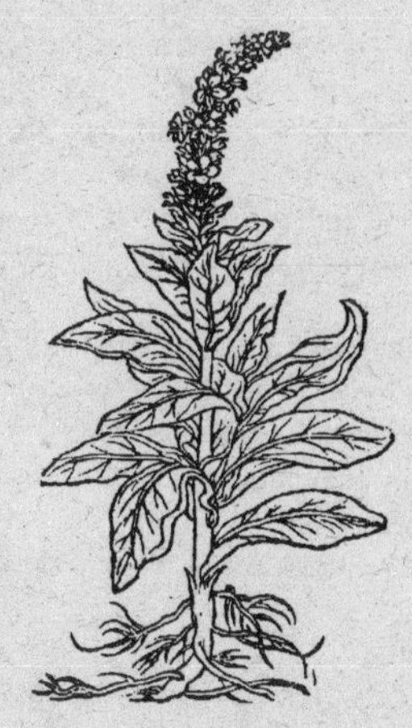

mullein

complaints, hoarseness, bronchitis, asthma, whooping-cough, wasting diseases and bleeding of the lungs and bowels. It can also be good for diarrhoea, mild catarrh, colic, inflammation of the urinary system, and as a poultice for boils and sores. The dried leaves may be smoked to remove irritation of the mucous membranes, the cough associated with consumption and spasmodic coughs in general. After placing bruised mullein leaves in olive oil and leaving it for a period, the oil can be used for relieving pain from bruises, frostbite and earache. Water distilled from the flowers was recommended for gout, burns and the condition called erysipelas, where the skin and tissue is infected with the bacterium *Streptococcus pyogenes* and the affected areas are red and swollen.

ADMINISTERED AS: fluid extract, distilled water, poultice, tincture, decoction.

Musk seed *Hibiscus abelmoschus.*

COMMON NAME: ambretta, Egyptian alcée, bisornkorner, target-leaved hibiscus, galu gastrin, *Abelmoschus moschatus.*

OCCURRENCE: native to India and grown in Egypt and the East and West Indies.

PARTS USED: the seeds. They contain fixed oil, a resin and a volatile body.

MEDICINAL USES: antispasmodic, aromatic, stomachic, nervine, aphrodisiac, insecticide. An emulsion of the seeds is regarded as antispasmodic and the seeds were chewed to benefit the nerves and stomach. The seeds are dusted over woollens to protect the fibre from moths.

ADMINISTERED AS: whole seeds, emulsion.

Mustard, Black *Brassica nigra, Siriapis nigra.*

COMMON NAME: *Brassica sinapioides.*

OCCURRENCE: it grows wild throughout Europe, South Siberia, Turkey and North Africa and is cultivated in England, Italy, Germany and the Netherlands as a condiment.

PARTS USED: the seeds which contain an acrid, volatile oil, an active principle, the glucoside sinigrin and the enzyme myrosin. When the seeds are crushed with water, these latter two chemicals come into contact and form oil of mustard.

MEDICINAL USES: irritant, stimulant, diuretic and emetic. Mainly used as a poultice to relieve acute local pain, e.g. pneumonia, bronchitis and other respiratory organ diseases. The herb draws blood to the skin surface, easing congestion of the organs, headaches, neuralgia and spasms. The oil of mustard is a powerful irritant and rubefacient when undiluted, but is very useful when dissolved in spirit for chilblains, rheumatism and colic. A hot infusion of the seed is a stimulating footbath and aids removal of colds or headaches. Mustard flour, when taken internally, can act as an emetic, aperient and alterative herb and may also cure hic-cups. It is also a very good antiseptic and sterilizing agent and deodorizer.

ADMINISTERED AS: poultice, infusion, essential oil, seed flour, leaves.

Myrrh *Commiphora molmol.*

COMMON NAME: *Balsamodendron myrrha*, *Commiphora myrrha* var. *molmol*, mira, morr.

OCCURRENCE: obtained from bushes in North-East Africa and in Arabia.

PARTS USED: the oleo-gum-resin which contains volatile oil, resins and gum.

MEDICINAL USES: stimulant, tonic, healing, antiseptic, astringent, expectorant, emmenagogue. Myrrh has a long history of use in countering poisons and putrid tissues throughout the body. It is used in leucorrhoea, chronic catarrh, thrush, athlete's foot, absence of menstrual periods, ulcers and as a vermifuge. The resin acts as a tonic in

dyspepsia, stimulates the circulation, appetite and the production of gastric juices. It makes a very good gargle or mouth-wash for an inflamed sore throat, spongy gums and mouth ulcers.
ADMINISTERED AS: fluid extract, tincture, pills.

Nettle *Urtica dioica, Urtica urens.*
COMMON NAME: common nettle, stinging nettle.
OCCURRENCE: widely distributed throughout temperate Europe and Asia, Japan, South Africa and Australia.
PARTS USED: the whole herb, which contains formic acid, mucilage, mineral salts, ammonia and carbonic acid.
MEDICINAL USES: astringent, stimulating, diuretic, tonic. The herb is anti-asthmatic and the juice of the nettle will relieve bronchial and asthmatic troubles, as will the dried leaves when burnt and inhaled. The seeds are taken as an infusion or in wine to ease consumption or ague. Nettles are used widely as a food source and can be made into puddings, tea, beer, juice and used as a vegetable. A hair tonic or lotion can also be made from the nettle. In the Highlands of Scotland, they were chopped, added to egg white and applied to the temples as a cure for insomnia.
ADMINISTERED AS: expressed juice, infusion, decoction, seeds, dried herb, dietary item.

Nightshade, Black *Solarum nignum.*
COMMON NAME: garden nightshade, petty morel.
OCCURRENCE: a common plant in south England, seen less frequently in northern England and Scotland.
PARTS USED: the whole plant, fresh leaves. Both contain the active principle, solanine which is found in variable quantities within the plant, throughout the year.
MEDICINAL USES: the bruised fresh leaves are used external to the body to ease pain and reduce inflammation. Juice of the leaves

has been used for ringworm, gout and earache and is supposed to make a good gargle or mouthwash when mixed with vinegar. This species of plant is reputed to be very poisonous, narcotic and sudorific, so is only utilized in very small doses, under careful supervision.
ADMINISTERED AS: infusion, expressed juice and fresh leaves.

Nutmeg *Myristica fragrans.*
COMMON NAME: nux moschata, *Myristica officinalis*, *M. aromata*, myristica.
OCCURRENCE: native to the Banda Islands, Malay Archipelago and the Molucca Islands. It is cultivated in Java, West Indies, Sumatra and French Guiana.
PARTS USED: the dried kernel of the seed which contains a volatile and a fixed oil, starch, gum, various acids and terpenes.
MEDICINAL USES: carminative, stomachic, stimulant. The grated or powdered kernel is used to relieve flatulence, vomiting and nausea. It is mainly used as an ingredient of various medicines and as a culinary spice. Nutmeg has similar properties to MACE but mace has a stronger flavour. Large doses of nutmeg can be toxic, producing disorientation, double vision and convulsions.
ADMINISTERED AS: expressed oil, powdered kernel.

Nux vomica *Strychnos Nux-vomica.*
COMMON NAME: poison nut, semen strychnox, Quaker buttons.
OCCURRENCE: a tree indigenous to India and now grown in Burma, China, Australia and the Malay Archipelago.
PARTS USED: the dried ripe seeds. They contain the alkaloids, strychnine, brucine and strychnicine, fatty matter, caffeotannic acid and the glucoside, loganin.
MEDICINAL USES: tonic, bitter, stimulant. Nux vomica is utilized as a general tonic, mainly when combined with other herbal remedies,

to treat neuralgia, dyspepsia, impotence, chronic constipation and general debility. This drug can also be of benefit in cardiac failure, surgical shock or poisoning by chloroform where it raises blood pressure and increases pulse rate, but it can also cause violent convulsions. Nux vomica should only be used in limited circumstances and under strict control as strychnine is very poisonous.
ADMINISTERED AS: fluid extract, tincture.

Oak *Quercus robur.*
COMMON NAME: common oak, tanner's bark.
OCCURRENCE: a tree widely dispersed over Europe.
PARTS USED: the bark.
MEDICINAL USES: slightly tonic, strongly astringent, antiseptic. It is very good in chronic diarrhoea, dysentery as a decoction and used as a gargle for sore throats. May also be used as an injection for leucorrhoea and applied locally for piles and bleeding gums. Water distilled from the oak buds was said to be good on any kind of inflammation.
ADMINISTERED AS: fluid extract, infusion, tincture, injection.

Oats *Avena sativa.*
COMMON NAME: groats, oatmeal.
OCCURRENCE: distributed across Europe, Britain and the USA.
PARTS USED: the seeds which are made up of starch, gluten, albumen and other proteins, sugar, gum oil and salts.
MEDICINAL USES: nervine, stimulant, antispasmodic, *Avena* forms a nutritious and easily digested food for convalescent patients and exhaustion after fevers. It can be made into a demulcent enema, or a good emollient poultice. Oat extract or tincture is useful as a nerve and uterine tonic.
ADMINISTERED AS: fluid extract, tincture, enema, dietary item.

Olive *Olea Europea.*
COMMON NAME: *Olea oleaster*, *Olea larcifolia*, *Olea gallica*, oliver.
OCCURRENCE: native to the Mediterranean countries, Syria and Turkey. Now cultivated in Chile, Peru and Australia.
PARTS USED: the oil expressed from the ripe fruit, the leaves.
MEDICINAL USES: the oil is emollient, demulcent, laxative and aperient. It is a good substitute for CASTOR OIL when given to children, but its value in clearing parasitic worms or gallstones is unsure. The oil is a good ingredient in liniments or ointment and is used for bruises, sprains, cutaneous injuries and rheumatic prob-lems. It is also utilized externally in joint, kidney and chest com-plaints or for chills, typhoid and scarlet fevers, plague and dropsy. When combined with alcohol, the oil is good as a hair tonic. Olive leaves have astringent and antiseptic properties, and an infusion of these leaves has proved beneficial in obstinate fevers.
ADMINISTERED AS: expressed oil, infusion, ointment.

Onion *Allium cepa.*
OCCURRENCE: originally native to south-west Asia and now cultivated around the globe.
PARTS USED: the bulb.
MEDICINAL USES: diuretic, expectorant, antiseptic. Although onions are extensively used in cookery, they also have medicinal uses. A roasted onion is applied to tumours or earache to remove the pain and onions steeped in gin produce a fluid extract which is given for gravel and dropsy. A homoeopathic remedy is made from red onions and

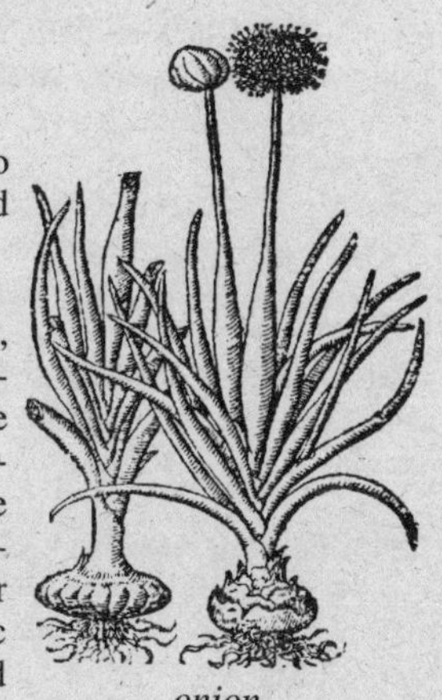

onion

is useful in neuralgic pain, colds, hay fever, toothache and in the early stages of laryngitis with hoarseness.
ADMINISTERED AS: poultice, tincture.

Orange, Bitter *Citrus aurantium* subsp. *amara*. **Orange, Sweet** *Citrus vulgaris*.
COMMON NAME: (bitter orange) *Citrus bigaradia*, *Citrus vulgaris*, *Bi garadier*, bigarade orange, Seville orange, naranja; (sweet orange) Portugal orange, China orange, *Citrus dulcis*.
OCCURRENCE: the bitter orange originated from northern India but is now grown in Mediterranean countries. The sweet orange is grown in Sicily, Africa and the West Indies.
PARTS USED: the fruit, peel and flowers. Oil is extracted from the peel of both types of orange—bitter orange produces oil of bigarde and the sweet orange oil is oil of Portugal. Distillation of the bitter orange flowers with water produces orange flower water and an essential oil called neroli.
MEDICINAL USES: tonic, stomachic, carminative, aromatic. Both sweet and bitter orange oils are used as flavouring agents for medicinal compounds but may be used in a similar manner to oil of TURPENTINE in treating chronic bronchitis. An infusion of dried flowers can be taken as a mild nervous stimulant and a tonic may be given of bitter orange peel, either on its own or as an infusion. In China, the dried peel of the sweet orange is used as a diuretic and to aid digestion. Oil of neroli is used in aromatherapy for treating anxiety and nervous depression.
ADMINISTERED AS: infusion, dried peel, essential oil, distilled water.

Orris *Iris florentina* (and other species).
COMMON NAME: Florentine orris, orris root.
OCCURRENCE: grown in Italy and Morocco and to a smaller extent in England.

PARTS USED: the root, which contains oil of orris, fat, resin, starch, mucilage, a glucoside called iridin and a bitter extractive substance.
MEDICINAL USES: Orris root is rarely used in medicine today. The fresh root has emetic, diuretic and cathartic properties and was formerly used against congested headache, dropsy, bronchitis and chronic diarrhoea. It is more generally used in perfumery, as it strengthens the odour of other fragrant herbs and acts as a fixative in perfumes and pot pourri. It is also part of dusting powders, toilet powders and tooth powders.

Paraguay Tea *Ilex paraguayensis.*
COMMON NAME: Paraguay herb, maté, yerba maté, jesuit's tea, Brazil tea, gón gouha, ilex maté, houx maté.
OCCURRENCE: largely cultivated in South America.
PARTS USED: the leaves, which contain caffeine, tannin ash and insoluble matter.
MEDICINAL USES: tonic, diuretic, diaphoretic, powerful stimulant. The leaves are infused in a similar manner to TEA and drunk with lemon juice and sugar by the local people in South America. There is a huge consumption of this herb as it is taken at every meal. In large doses, it can cause purging and vomiting.
ADMINISTERED AS: infusion.

Paris, Herb *Paris quadrifolia.*
COMMON NAME: herba Paris, true love, one berry, *Solarum quadrifolium, Aconitum pardalianches.*
OCCURRENCE: found in Europe, Russian Asia and locally distributed in Great Britain.
PARTS USED: the whole plant picked as it is just coming into bloom.
MEDICINAL USES: narcotic. In large doses, the herb induces nausea, vertigo, vomiting, profuse sweating, delirium, dry throat and con-

vulsions. Overdoses can be fatal, particularly in children. If administered in small doses, the herb can relieve spasmodic cough, rheumatism, bronchitis, cramp, heart palpitation and colic. Juice expressed from the leaves is good for green wounds, tumours and inflammation while the juice from the berries eases inflammation of the eyes. In Russia, the leaves are proposed to ease madness and its effects. As it has a similar set of qualities to opium, it has been used as an aphrodisiac. Herb Paris has also been utilized as an antidote against mercury and arsenic poisoning.
ADMINISTERED AS: tincture, expressed juice of leaves, expressed juice of berries, ointment, powdered root, decoction.

Parsley *Carum petroselinum.*
COMMON NAME: *Apium petroselinum*, *Petroselinum lativum*, petersylinge, persely, persele.
OCCURRENCE: this was first cultivated in Britain in 1548, now completely naturalized through England and Scotland.
PARTS USED: the root, seeds and leaves. The root is slightly aromatic and contains starch mucilage, sugar, volatile oil and apiin. Parsley seeds contain more volatile oil, which consists of terpenes and apiol, an allyl compound.
MEDICINAL USES: carminative, tonic, aperient, diuretic. A strong decoction of the root is used in gravel, stone, kidney congestion, jaundice and dropsy. Bruised parsley seeds used to be given against plague and intermittent fevers, while the external application of the leaves may help to dispel tumours. A poultice of the leaves is effective against bites and stings of poisonous insects.
ADMINISTERED AS: fluid extract, essential oil, infusion, ointment and poultice.

Parsley piert *Alchemilla arvensis.*
COMMON NAME: parsley breakstone, parsley piercestone, field lady's mantle.
OCCURRENCE: common across Great Britain, Europe and North Africa and was introduced into North America.
PARTS USED: the herb.
MEDICINAL USES: diuretic, demulcent, refrigerant. This herb is mainly employed in gravel, stone, dropsy and in bladder and kidney problems. It can effect results even in seemingly incurable cases. It can also help jaundice and clearing obstructions of the liver. To limit its irritancy, it is sometimes combined with demulcent or diuretic herbs for best effect, e.g. BROOM, JUNIPER, CARROT, COMFREY or MARSHMALLOW.
ADMINISTERED AS: fresh herb or infusion.

Parsnip *Pastinaca sativa.*
COMMON NAME: le panais, die pastinake.
OCCURRENCE: native European, cultivated commercially as food.
PARTS USED: the root.
MEDICINAL USES: nutritive. The parsnip exceeds almost all other vegetables in terms of food value (except potatoes) and is very nourishing for humans and animals alike. They are preferred to carrots for fattening pigs and given to cattle. Some old herbalists saw parsnips as a cure for asthma, cancer and consumption and used bruised parsnip roots as an application on bruises. In many areas, parsnips were made into a preserve, a beer or wine. They are also used extensively in salads, soups, as a vegetable and in cakes.

Passionflower *Passiflora incarnata.*
COMMON NAME: passion vine, granadilla, maracoc, maypops.
OCCURRENCE: a native of Virginia in the United States.
PARTS USED: the flower and the dried vine. The plant contains

flavonoids, sugars, sterols and gum as well as the alkaloids harmone, harmol, harmaline, harmine and harmalol.
MEDICINAL USES: antispasmodic, sedative, narcotic. This drug relaxes the nervous system and the sedative effects are good as well. It is non-addictive. It is a very good remedy for anxiety, tension, insomnia, diarrhoea, dysentery, neuralgia and painful menstruation. The alkaloids have tranquillizing effects and it is used to reduce high blood pressure.
ADMINISTERED AS: fluid extract.

Peach *Prunus persica.*
COMMON NAME: *Persica vulgaris, Amygdalus persica.*
OCCURRENCE: cultivated in Asia for centuries and introduced into Europe from Persia.
PARTS USED: the bark, leaves and the oil expressed from the weeds.
MEDICINAL USES: demulcent, sedative, diuretic, expectorant. The leaves or bark, when used as an infusion, are almost a specific for irritation and congestion of the gastric surfaces. The infusion is also good for chronic bronchitis, whooping cough and ordinary coughs. A syrup or infusion made of the peach flowers was thought to be a mild acting purgative for children, as well as good for jaundice and giving health to a poorly child. The kernel oil was thought to induce sleep and rest if rubbed on to the temples. The oil is also used as a substitute for the more expensive ALMOND oil.
ADMINISTERED AS: infusion, fresh leaves, powdered leaves, oil.

Pellitory *Anacyclus pyrethrum.*
COMMON NAME: Roman pellitory, pellitory of Spain, Spanish chamomile, pyrethre, *Matricaria pyrethrum, Anthemis pyrethrum, Pyrethrum officinarum, Pyrethri radix.*
OCCURRENCE: cultivated in Spain, Algeria and other Mediterranean countries.

PARTS USED: the root, which contains two oils, a brown resin thought to contain peletonin, tannin, gum, lignin and various mineral salts. The alkaloid, pyrethrine is the active chemical.
MEDICINAL USES: local irritant, rubefacient. The main use of this herb is to relieve toothache and promoting the flow of saliva. This eases conditions such as dryness of the throat and partial paralysis of the lips and tongue. The powdered root is used as snuff to clear chronic catarrh of the head, exciting the flow of nasal mucous and tears. The herb is added to many dental toothpowders.
ADMINISTERED AS: powdered root, infusion, tincture.

Pellitory-of-the-wall *Parietaria officinalis.*
COMMON NAME: *Parietaria diffusa*, lichwort, paritary.
OCCURRENCE: a common wild plant in Europe and Great Britain.
PARTS USED: the herb, which contains a bitter glucoside, tannin, sulphur, mucilage and flavones among its chemical constituents.
MEDICINAL USES: diuretic, laxative, refrigerant, demulcent. It is given as an infusion or decoction to treat urine retention, cystitis, nephritis, dropsy, prostate inflammation, urinary stones and gravel. In the form of an ointment, this herb was used for haemorrhoids, gout and fistulas. The fresh herb is more effective than the dried herb.
ADMINISTERED AS: infusion, syrup, poultice, decoction.

Pennyroyal *Mentha pulegium.*
COMMON NAME: pulegium, run-by-the-ground, pudding grass, lurk-in-the-ditch, piliolerial.
OCCURRENCE: a native plant of most of Europe and parts of Asia and commonly grown in gardens.
PARTS USED: the herb and the oil distilled from the herb called oil of pulegiam.

Medicinal uses: carminative, diaphoretic, stimulant, emmenagogue. The herb is mainly used to bring on menstruation which has been obstructed by cold or chills. It is also beneficial in spasms, flatulence, hysteria, sickness, colds, headaches and is a blood purifying herb. Pennyroyal is supposed to encourage sleep and was hung in bedrooms for that purpose. The oil has been used to prevent mosquito and gnat bites for many years. If taken internally, the oil can be highly toxic and death can result. This herb should not be taken by pregnant women as it promotes menstruation and may cause haemorrhage and death.
Administered as: dried herb, infusion, distilled oil.

Peony *Paeonia officinalis.*
Common name: paeony, paeonia, common peony, piney, *Paeonia lactifloria, Paeonia corrallina.*
Occurrence: introduced into Great Britain some centuries ago.
Parts used: the root, which contains benzoic acid, asparagin, an alkaloid and an essential oil.
Medicinal uses: antispasmodic, tonic. In the past, peony has been used successfully in spasmodic nervous problems such as epilepsy and spasms as well as lunacy. An infusion of the powdered root is recommended for liver obstructions, and helps kidney and gall bladder diseases. Since this plant is poisonous, it is rarely utilized in modern herbal medicine.
Administered as: infusion.

Pepper *Piper nigrum.*
Common name: black pepper, piper.
Occurrence: grows wild in South India and Cechin-China; now cultivated in the East and West Indies, Malay Archipelago, the Philippines, Java, Sumatra and Borneo.
Parts used: the dried unripe fruits. White pepper comes from the

same plant, except that the pericarp of the fruit has been removed prior to drying. The active chemicals in black or white pepper are piperine, volatile oil, starch, cellulose and a resin called chavicin.
MEDICINAL USES: aromatic, stimulant, carminative, febrifuge. The herb is useful in treating constipation, gonorrhoea, prolapsed rectum, paralysis of the tongue and acts on the urinary organs. The stimulant properties of pepper work on the gastro-intestinal system to aid digestion, ease dyspepsia, torbid stomach conditions, and relieve flatulence and nausea. Pepper has also been recommended in diarrhoea, cholera, scarlatina, vertigo and paralytic and arthritic disorders. Peppercorns, as the dried fruit is known, are used both whole and ground in many culinary dishes and are used as a condiment. In the Siege of Rome in 408 AD, pepper was so highly priced that it was used as a form of currency.
ADMINISTERED AS: powdered dried fruits, gargle.

Peppermint *Mentha piperita.*
COMMON NAME: brandy mint, curled mint, balm mint.
OCCURRENCE: found across Europe, was introduced into Britain and grows widely in damp places and waste ground.
PARTS USED: the herb and distilled oil. The plant contains peppermint oil, which is composed of menthol, menthyl acetate and isovalerate, menthone, cineol, pinene and limonene. The medicinal qualities are found in the alcoholic chemicals.
MEDICINAL USES: stimulant, antispasmodic, carminative, stomachic, oil of peppermint is extensively used in both medicine and commerce. It is good in dyspepsia, flatulence, colic and abdominal cramps. The oil allays sickness and nausea, is used for chorea and diarrhoea but is normally used with other medicines to disguise unpalatable tastes and effects. Peppermint water is in most general use and is used to raise body temperature and in-

duce perspiration. Peppermint tea can help ward off colds and influenza at an early stage, can calm heart palpitations and is used to reduce the appetite.
ADMINISTERED AS: infusion, distilled water, spirit, essential oil and fluid extract.

Pimpernel, Scarlet *Anagallis arvensis*.

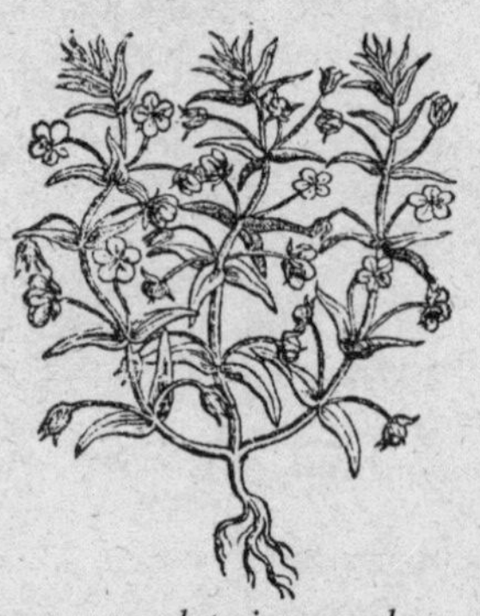

scarlet pimpernel

COMMON NAME: shepherd's barometer, poor man's weatherglass, adder's eyes, bipinella.
OCCURRENCE: a very widely distributed plant found in all the temperate regions, in both hemispheres.
PARTS USED: the whole herb, of which little is known of the active chemicals within it. It does contain the compound, saponin.
MEDICINAL USES: diuretic, diaphoretic, expectorant. This plant has an ancient reputation for healing, particularly dealing with diseases of the brain and mental illness. It is considered beneficial in dropsy, liver obstruction, disorders of the spleen, gravel, rheumatic complaints and gout, but caution should be taken as in experiments extracts from this plant have been found to be poisonous to animals and its full effects on humans are not yet known.
ADMINISTERED AS: infusion, dried herb, tincture, fluid extract.

Pine oils there are several kinds: **Siberian pine oil**, from *Abies Sibirica*; **Pumilio pine oil**, from *Pinus muge*; **Sylvestris pine oil**, from *Pinus sylvestris*.

PARTS USED: the oil produced from when pine wood is distilled using steam under pressure.
MEDICINAL USES: rubefacient, aromatic. These oils are mainly used as inhalants for bronchitis or laryngitis or as liniment plasters.
ADMINISTERED AS: distilled oil.

Pine, White *Pinus strobus.*
COMMON NAME: Weymouth pine, pin du lord, *Pinus alba*, deal pine.
OCCURRENCE: widely distributed in the northern hemisphere, especially in North America.
PARTS USED: the bark.
MEDICINAL USES: expectorant, diuretic, demulcent. Used for the relief of coughs, colds and chest diseases. It has a beneficial effect on the bladder and kidney systems. A compound syrup is the most commonly administered form of the drug, but it contains morphine so care must be taken that morphine dependence does not develop.
ADMINISTERED AS: compound syrup and fluid extract.

Pink root *Spigelia marylandica.*
COMMON NAME: Indian pink, wormgrass, carolina pink, Maryland pink, American wormroot, starbloom.
OCCURRENCE: grows in the southern states of the United States of America.
PARTS USED: the whole plant or the root. This plant contains a poisonous alkaloid called spigeline, volatile oil, resin, mucilage, lignin, a bitter principle and salts of calcium potassium and sodium.
MEDICINAL USES: very active vermifuge. This plant has very beneficial effects on removing tapeworms and roundworms, and is safe enough to give to children as long as a saline aperient is given after pinkroot, to temper the unpleasant side effects. These

side effects include disturbed vision, muscular spasms, increased heart action and dizziness and are increased in severity as the dose given rises. This can lead to convulsions and death if care is not taken with this drug.
ADMINISTERED AS: fluid extract, powdered root.

Pipsissewa *Chinaphila umbellata.*
COMMON NAME: winter green, butter winter, prince's pine, king's cure, ground holly, love in winter, rheumatism weed, *Pyrola umbellata.*
OCCURRENCE: grows in Europe, Asia, the United States and Siberia.
PARTS USED: the leaves, which contain chinaphilin, arbutin gum, resin, pectic acid, starch, chlorophyll, tannic acids and several mineral salts.
MEDICINAL USES: diuretic, astringent, tonic, alterative. A decoction of the leaves is good for fluid retention, chronic gonorrhoea, dropsy and catarrh of the bladder. Applied to the skin, it acts as a rubefacient and vesicant which is good in kidney and cardiac diseases, scrofular and chronic rheumatism. It is also of value in skin diseases and may be a effective against diabetes.
ADMINISTERED AS: fresh leaves, decoction, fluid extract, syrup.

Plantain, Common *Plantago major.*
COMMON NAME: broad-leaved plantain, ripple grass, waybread, snakeweed, cuckoo's bread, Englishman's foot, white man's foot, waybroad.
OCCURRENCE: a familiar weed all over Europe, Great Britain and other parts of the world.
PARTS USED: the root, leaves and flowers.
MEDICINAL USES: refrigerant, diuretic, deobstruent, astringent, cooling, alterative. The plant has been used in inflammation of the skin, malignant ulcers, intermittent fever, applied to sores and as

a vulnerary. The fresh leaves can stop bleeding of minor wounds, relieve the pain of insect stings, nettles, burns and scalds.

ADMINISTERED AS: expressed juice, poultice, infusion, fresh leaves, fluid extract, decoction, ointment.

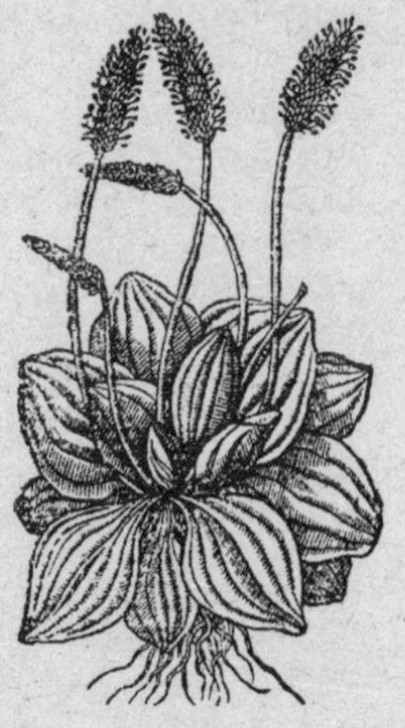

plantain

Pleurisy root *Asclepias tuberose.*

COMMON NAME: butterfly-weed, swallow-wort, tuber root, wind root, colic root, orange milkweed, white root, flux root, Canada root.

OCCURRENCE: native to North America.

PARTS USED: the root which contains several resins, volatile oil, fatty matter, glucosides including asclepiadin and cardiac glycosides.

MEDICINAL USES: antispasmodic, diaphoretic, expectorant, tonic, carminative, mildly cathartic. One of the most important indigenous North American herbs which has a specific action on the lungs, reducing inflammation, helping expectoration and delivering a mild tonic effect to the pulmonary system. It is of great benefit in pleurisy, pulmonary catarrh and difficult breathing as it relieves the pain. The root also helps in acute and chronic rheumatism, eczema, flatulent colic, indigestion, dysentery and diarrhoea. It is often combined with other herbs, e.g. ANGELICA to best effect. In large doses, pleurisy root can be emetic and purgative in effect.

ADMINISTERED AS: decoction, fluid extract, infusion.

Poke root *Phytolacca decandra.*

COMMON NAME: garget, pigeon berry, bear's grape, red-ink plant,

American spinach, skoke, crowberry, cancer-root, pocan, coakum, poke berry, herbe de la laque, *Phytolaccae radix*, *Phytolacca vulgaris*, *P. americana*, *Blitun americanum*.
OCCURRENCE: indigenous to North America and is grown in most Mediterranean countries.
PARTS USED: dried root and berries. The root is made up of triterpenoid saponins, phytolaccine (an alkaloid), resins, phytolaccic acid and tannin.
MEDICINAL USES: emetic, cathartic, alterative, narcotic. The root is used for conjunctivitis, chronic rheumatism, skin diseases and paralysis of the bowels. It is said to stimulate the lymphatic system and so is good for tonsillitis, swollen glands and mumps. Herbalists disagree as to whether poke root is effective against cancer. It may be effective, when used both as a poultice and taken internally, against breast cancer and mastitis and has been used in cases of uterine cancer. The berries are thought to have a milder action on the body than the root. The use of the root as an emetic is not recommended and the fresh root is poisonous so this drug should only be prescribed by a qualified herbal practitioner.
ADMINISTERED AS: infusion, ointment, tincture, fluid extract.

Polypody root *Polypodium vulgare*.
COMMON NAME: rock polypody, polypody of the oak, wall fern, brake root, rock brake, oak fern, rock of polypody.
OCCURRENCE: a common fern growing in sheltered places, hedgebanks, old walls and tree stumps in Great Britain and Europe.
PARTS USED: the root.
MEDICINAL USES: alterative, tonic, expectorant, pectoral. This herb is used as a laxative; as a tonic in dyspepsia and loss of appetite. It is also good for skin diseases, coughs and catarrh, consumption, hepatic complaints and some types of parasitic worm. The action of this drug is such that it may cause the formation of a

rash, but these spots should disappear after a short period of time with no after effects. This fern is still used as a cure for whooping cough in many rural areas.
ADMINISTERED AS: fresh root, decoction, powdered root, fluid extract.

Poplar *Populus tremuloides.*
COMMON NAME: white poplar, American aspen, quaking aspen.
OCCURRENCE: native to North America and commonly grown in Great Britain.
PARTS USED: the bark, which is thought to contain salicin and populin.
MEDICINAL USES: febrifuge, diuretic, stimulant, tonic. This drug is very useful against fevers, particularly those of an intermittent nature. It is often used as a substitute for PERUVIAN BARK or quinine, as it lacks dangerous long-term side effects. Poplar bark is helpful in treating chronic diarrhoea, debility, hysteria, indigestion and faintness as well as acting as a diuretic in gleet, gonorrhoea and urinary complaints. This drug could be considered a 'universal tonic'.
ADMINISTERED AS: infusion, fluid extract.

Poppy, Red *Papaver rhoeas.*
COMMON NAME: headache, corn poppy, corn rose, flores rhoeados.
OCCURRENCE: a common flowering plant in fields and waste ground across Europe and Great Britain.
PARTS USED: flowers and petals. the fresh petals contain rhoeadic and papaveric acids, which give the flowers their colour, and the alkaloid rhoeadine. The amount and quantity of active ingredients in the plant is uncertain so its action is open to debate.
MEDICINAL USES: very slightly narcotic, anodyne, expectorant. The petals can be made into a syrup which is used to ease pain. It may be used for chest complaints, e.g. pleurisy.
ADMINISTERED AS: syrup, infusion, distilled water.

Poppy, White *Papaver somniferum.*
COMMON NAME: opium poppy, mawseed.
OCCURRENCE: indigenous to Turkey and Asia, cultivated in Europe, Great Britain, Persia, India and China for opium production.
PARTS USED: the capsules and flowers. The white poppy contains twenty one different alkaloids of which morphine, narcotine, codeine, codamine and thebaine are the most important.
MEDICINAL USES: hypnotic, sedative, astringent, expectorant, diaphoretic, antispasmodic, anodyne. The use of this drug dates back to Greek and Roman times. It is the best possible hypnotic and sedative drug, frequently used to relieve pain and calm excitement. It has also been used in diarrhoea, dysentery and some forms of cough. The tincture of opium is commonly called laudanum, and when applied externally with soap liniment it provides quick pain relief.
ADMINISTERED AS: syrup, tincture, decoction and poultice.

Primrose *Primula vulgaris.*
OCCURRENCE: a common wild flower found in woods, hedgerows and pastures throughout Great Britain.
PARTS USED: the root and whole herb. Both parts of the plant contain a fragrant oil called primulin and the active principle saponin.
MEDICINAL USES: astringent, antispasmodic, vermifuge, emetic. It was formerly considered to be an important remedy in muscular rheumatism, paralysis and gout. A tincture of the whole plant has sedative effects and is used successfully in extreme sensitivity, restlessness and insomnia. Nervous headaches can be eased by treatment with an infusion of the root, while the powdered dry root serves as an emetic. An infusion of primrose flowers is excellent in nervous headaches and an ointment can be made out of the leaves to heal and salve wounds and cuts.
ADMINISTERED AS: infusion, tincture, powdered root and ointment.

Puffball *Lycoperdon bovista.*
COMMON NAME: *Lycoperdon giganteum.*
OCCURRENCE: grows wild throughout Great Britain and Europe.
PARTS USED: the lower section of the fungi.
MEDICINAL USES: haemostatic. This fungi grows completely enclosing its spores in fungal tissue (peridium), and then matures so that the colour changes from yellow-white to brown and then the peridium ruptures and the spores are released. When young, the spongy fungal tissue makes an excellent food and is consumed with relish by people in many European areas, including the Gaelic community in the Highlands of Scotland. Once matured, it is not edible but it can then be used to stop bleeding from wounds. It is a highly effective cure. Puffballs were also used as tinder many years ago and are burnt, producing smoke which stupefies bees so that honey can be collected safely.
ADMINISTERED AS: dried or fresh fungal tissue and spores.

Pumpkin *Cucurbita maxima.*
COMMON NAME: pumpkin seed, melon pumpkin, pompion.
OCCURRENCE: a plant grown for food and animal fodder in the United States and common in gardens in Great Britain.
PARTS USED: the seeds. They contain a fixed oil, a volatile oil, sugar, starch and an acrid resin which may be the active component.
MEDICINAL USES: taeniacide, diuretic, demulcent. This fruit has long been used as a vermifuge, removing parasitic worms including tapeworm. A mixture of the seeds, sugar, milk or water is mixed up and taken over six hours after which CASTOR OIL is given, a few hours after the final dose of pumpkin. The vermifuge effects are thought to come from the mechanical effects of the seeds. A basic infusion of the seeds in water is used in urinary complaints.
ADMINISTERED AS: infusion.

Purslane, Golden *Portulaca sativa.*
COMMON NAME: garden purslane, pigweed.
OCCURRENCE: an herbaceous annual plant which is distributed all over the world. It is not indigenous to Great Britain.
PARTS USED: the herb, expressed juice and seeds.
MEDICINAL USES: Purslane is a herb with a great history of use for medical complaints. The expressed juice of the herb was good for strangury, dry coughs, shortness of breath, hot agues, headaches, stopping haemorrhages and as an external application to sores and inflammation. When combined with oil of ROSES, the juice was used for sore mouths, swollen gums and to fasten loose teeth. The bruised seeds were made into a decoction with wine and used to expel worms from children. The bruised herb was used as a poultice to remove heat from the head and temples and to reduce eye inflammation. It was also used on cramps or gouty areas.
ADMINISTERED AS: poultice, decoction, expressed juice.

Pyrethrum, Dalmatian *Chrysanthemum cinerariaefolium.*
COMMON NAME: insect flowers.
OCCURRENCE: the Dalmatian coast and Japan.
PARTS USED: the closed flowers.
MEDICINAL USES: insecticide, vermin killer. A powder of ground flowers is used in powder, lotions and fumigation materials to kill insects. The active ingredient is pyrethrin. The powder is not toxic to mammals.
ADMINISTERED AS: ground flowers.

Quince *Cydonia oblongata.*
COMMON NAME: quince seed, *Cydonica vulgaris.*
OCCURRENCE: grown in England for its fruit but is native to Persia.
PARTS USED: the fruit and seeds.

MEDICINAL USES: astringent, mucilaginous, demulcent. The fruit is used to prepare a syrup which is added to drinks when ill, as it restrains looseness of the bowels and helps relieve dysentery and diarrhoea. The soaked seeds form a mucilaginous mass similar to that produced by FLAX. A decoction of the seeds is used against gonorrhoea, thrush and in irritable conditions of the mucous membranes. The liquid is also used as a skin lotion or cream and administered in eye diseases as a soothing lotion.
ADMINISTERED AS: syrup, decoction or lotion.

Radish *Raphanus satinus.*
OCCURRENCE: a native plant of China, Japan and Vietnam and widely cultivated in Europe, Great Britain and temperate Asia.
PARTS USED: the root, which has been found to contain a volatile oil, an amylclytic enzyme and a chemical called phenylethyl isothiocyanite.
MEDICINAL USES: antiscorbutic, diuretic. This plant is a very good food remedy for scurvy, gravel and stone. The juice has been beneficial in preventing the formation of gallstones.
ADMINISTERED AS: expressed juice, fresh root, dietary item.

Ragwort *Senecio jacobaea.*
COMMON NAME: St. James's wort, stinking nanny, staggerwort, ragweed, dog standard, cankerwort, stammerwort, fireweed.
OCCURRENCE: an abundant wild plant, widely distributed over Great Britain, Europe, Siberia and north-west India.
PARTS USED: the herb.
MEDICINAL USES: diaphoretic, detergent, emollient, cooling, astringent. The leaves were used as emollient poultices, while the expressed juice of the herb was utilized as a wash in burns, eye inflammation, sores and cancerous ulcers. It has been successful in relieving rheumatism, sciatica, gout and in reducing inflamma-

tion and swelling of joints when applied as a poultice. Ragwort makes a good gargle for ulcerated throats and mouths and a decoction of its root is said to help internal bruising and wounds. The herb was previously thought to be able to prevent infection. This plant is poisonous to cattle and should be removed from their pastures. The alkaloids in the ragwort have cumulative effects in the cattle and low doses of the chemical eaten over a period of time can built up to a critical level, where the cattle show obvious symptoms and death then results. It is uncertain if sheep are also susceptible to this chemical.
ADMINISTERED AS: poultice, infusion and decoction.

Raspberry *Rubus idaeus*.
COMMON NAME: American raspberry, raspbis, hindberry, bramble of Mount Ida, *Rubus strigosus*.
OCCURRENCE: found wild in Great Britain and cultivated in many parts of Europe.
PARTS USED: the leaves and fruit. The fruit contains fruit sugar, a volatile oil, pectin, mineral salts and citric and malic acids.
MEDICINAL USES: astringent and stimulant. Tea made of raspberry leaves is employed as a gargle for sore mouths, canker of the throat and as a wash for wounds and ulcers. It was also reckoned to give strength to pregnant women and encourage fast and safe delivery of the child. The leaves make a good poultice for cleaning wounds and promoting healing. Raspberry vinegar made with fruit juice, sugar and white wine vinegar makes a very good cooling drink when added to water, and is beneficial in fevers and as a gargle for sore throats. The infusion of raspberry leaves is also good in extreme laxity of the bowels and in stomach complaints of children.
ADMINISTERED AS: infusion, poultice, tea and liquid extract.

Red root *Ceanothus americanus.*
COMMON NAME: New Jersey tea, wild snowball.
OCCURRENCE: a shrub indigenous to the United States.
PARTS USED: the root, which contains tannin, a resin, a bitter extract, gum, lignin, a volatile substance and a principle called ceanothine.
MEDICINAL USES: antispasmodic, astringent, expectorant, sedative, anti-syphilis drug. It is very good in chronic bronchitis, whooping cough, consumption, asthma, dysentery and pulmonary complaints. The decoction is an excellent mouth wash or gargle for sores or ulcers. The herb is also used as an injection for gonorrhoea, gleet and leucorrhoea.
ADMINISTERED AS: fluid extract, decoction, injection.

Rest-harrow *Ononis arvensis.*
COMMON NAME: wild liquorice, cammock, stinking tommy, ground furze, land whin, *Ononis spinosa.*
OCCURRENCE: a weed found on arable and waste land in Britain.
PARTS USED: the root.
MEDICINAL USES: diuretic. This herb was taken internally for dropsy, jaundice, gout, rheumatism and bladder stones. When made into a decoction, it was used as a wash for ulcers, fluid accumulation in tissues and enlarged glands. It was also proposed to subdue delirium. The young shoots were used as a vegetable or pickled, when they were said to refresh the breath and remove the smell of alcohol from the breath.
ADMINISTERED AS: decoction, dietary item.

Rhubarb, English *Rheum rhaponticum.*
COMMON NAME: garden rhubarb, bastard rhubarb, sweet round-leaved dock, *Rheum officinale.*
OCCURRENCE: its cultivation started in England around 1777 and

spread throughout Great Britain. It is found growing wild or near dwellings.

PARTS USED: the rhizome and root. The stem and leaves of the plant contain potassium oxalate in quantity and some people are more sensitive to these salts and should avoid eating the plant. People with gout or those subject to urinary irritation should avoid the plant as well.

MEDICINAL USES: stomachic, aperient, astringent, purgative. This plant has a milder action than its relative, Turkey rhubarb (*Rheum palmatum*). It has a milder purgative effect and is particularly useful for stomach troubles in infants and looseness of the bowels. In large doses, rhubarb has a laxative effect. A decoction of the seed is proposed to ease stomach pain and increase the appetite. Rhubarb leaves were formerly used as a vegetable in the nineteenth century, and several fatal cases of poisoning were recorded.

ADMINISTERED AS: decoction and powdered root.

Rice *Oryza sativa.*

COMMON NAME: nivona, dhan, bras, paddy, *Oryza montana*, *O. setegera*, *O. latifolia.*

OCCURRENCE: native to China and India; now cultivated in most sub-tropical countries.

PARTS USED: the seeds.

MEDICINAL USES: nutritive, demulcent, refrigerant. Boiled rice is good in treating upset digestion, bowel problems and diarrhoea. Rice-water, made from a decoction of the seeds, is an excellent demulcent and refrigerant drink in febrile and inflammatory diseases of the intestines, painful urination and other related conditions. It may be given as an enema for best results. Finely powdered rice flour can be used for burns, scalds and erysipelas or rice starch can be utilized in the same manner as wheat starch.

ADMINISTERED AS: poultice, decoction, dietary item, enema.

Rose, pale *Rosa centifolia.*
COMMON NAME: cabbage rose, hundred-leaved rose.
OCCURRENCE: cultivated in southern Europe and grown as a garden plant in many countries.
PARTS USED: the petals, which contain an acid red colouring matter, the glucoside quercitrin, gallic acid, tannic acid, sugar, gum and fat. Also the leaves.
MEDICINAL USES: aperient, laxative, astringent. The petals of this pink rose are rarely taken internally in modern herbal medicine, although they do have aperient properties. These flowers are mainly used for the preparation of rose-water, which is used as an eye lotion and as a carrier medium for other medicines. Cold cream is also made from rose-water and it is used on the skin of the hand and face to soothe abrasions and lesions. Rose leaves are laxative and astringent and were used to heal wounds.
ADMINISTERED AS: distilled water, ointment.

Rose, red *Rosa gallica.*
COMMON NAME: rose flowers, Provence rose, provins rose.
OCCURRENCE: a native plant of southern Europe and grown in gardens all over the world.
PARTS USED: the petals. Their composition is the same as that of the PALE ROSE, except they do not contain tannic acid.
MEDICINAL USES: tonic, astringent. Today, the petals are not normally taken internally. The petals are prepared in three manners which are then used. A confection is made of petals and sugar and this is utilized in making pills. The fluid extract is prepared using powdered rose petals, glycerine and dilute alcohol while an acid infusion is made with dried rose petals, sulphuric acid, sugar and boiling water. The infusion may be used as a flavouring for other medicines, as a lotion for eye complaints and for the treatment of night sweats relating to depression. Syrup of roses, honey of rose

and rose vinegar are also preparations used medicinally in various countries around Europe. The petals are also used as flavour enhancers in two alcoholic liqueurs. *Rosa gallica* petals are used in aromatherapy.
ADMINISTERED AS: pills, lotion, infusion, poultice, syrup, fluid extract.

Rosemary *Rosmarinus officinalis.*
COMMON NAME: polar plant, compass-weed, compass plant, romero, *Rosmarinus coronarium.*
OCCURRENCE: native to the dry hills of the Mediterranean, from Spain westward to Turkey. A common garden plant in Britain, having been cultivated prior to the Norman Conquest.
PARTS USED: the herb and root. Oil of rosemary is distilled from the plant tops and used medicinally. Rosemary contains tannic acid, a bitter principle, resin and a volatile oil.
MEDICINAL USES: tonic, astringent, diaphoretic, stimulant. The essential oil is also stomachic, nervine and carminative and cures many types of headache. It is mainly applied externally as a hair lotion which is said to prevent baldness and the formation of dandruff. The oil is used externally as a rubefacient and is added to liniments for fragrance and stimulant properties. Rosemary tea can remove headache, colic, colds and nervous diseases and may also lift nervous depression.
ADMINISTERED AS: infusion, essential oil and lotion.

Rosinweed *Silphium paciniatum.*
COMMON NAME: compass plant, compass-weed, polar plant.
OCCURRENCE: native to the western United States, especially Ohio. This plant is closely related to *Silphium laciniatum* and is often confused with it.
PARTS USED: the root, which yields a resinous secretion very similar to MASTIC.

MEDICINAL USES: tonic, diaphoretic, alterative, emetic, diuretic, antispasmodic, expectorant. The root is used in dry, stubborn coughs, asthma and other pulmonary diseases. The decoction of the root is said to be emetic and has cured intermittent fevers. A strong infusion is good against enlarged spleen, internal bruising, liver problems and digestive ulcers. The resin has diuretic qualities and taints the urine, giving it a strong odour.
ADMINISTERED AS: fluid extract, decoction, infusion.

Rowan tree *Pyrus aucuparia.*
COMMON NAME: mountain ash, *Sorbus aucuparia*, *Mespilus aucuparia.*
OCCURRENCE: generally distributed over Great Britain and Europe, especially at high altitudes.
PARTS USED: the bark and fruit. The fruit may contain tartaric, citric or malic acids dependent upon its stage of ripeness. It also contains sorbitol, sorbin, sorbit, parascorbic acid and bitter, acrid colouring matters. The bark contains amygdalin.
MEDICINAL USES: astringent, antiscorbutic. A decoction of Rowan bark is given for diarrhoea and as a vaginal injection for leucorrhoea. The berries are made into an acid gargle to ease sore throats and inflamed tonsils. An infusion of the fruit is administered to ease haemorrhoids. The berries may also be made into jelly, flour, cider, ale or an alcoholic spirit. The rowan tree planted next to a house was said to protect the house against witchcraft.
ADMINISTERED AS: decoction, injection, infusion and dietary item.

Rue *Ruta graveolens.*
COMMON NAME: herb of grace, garden rue, herbygrass, ave-grace.
OCCURRENCE: indigenous to southern Europe and was introduced into Great Britain by the Romans.
PARTS USED: the herb. The herb is covered by glands which contain

a volatile oil. The oil is composed of methylnonylketone, limonene, cineole, a crystalline substance called rutin and several acids. The plant also contains several alkaloids including fagarine and arborinine as well as coumarins.
MEDICINAL USES: stimulant, antispasmodic, emmenagogue, irritant, rubefacient. This is a very powerful herb and the dose administered should be kept low. It is useful in treating coughs, croup, colic, flatulence, hysteria and it is particularly good against strained eyes and headaches caused by eyestrain. An infusion of the herb is good for nervous indigestion, heart palpitations, nervous headaches and to expel worms. The chemical, rutin, strengthens weak blood vessels and aids varicose veins. In Chinese medicine, rue is a specific for insect and snake bites. When made into an ointment, rue is effective in gouty and rheumatic pains, sprained and bruised tendons and chilblains. The bruised leaves irritate and blister the skin and so can ease sciatica. This herb should not be used in pregnancy as the volatile oil, alkaloids and coumarins in the plant all stimulate the uterus and strongly promote menstrual bleeding. When a fresh leaf is chewed, it flavours the mouth and relieves headache, giddiness or any hysterical spasms quickly.
ADMINISTERED AS: fresh leaf, volatile oil, ointment, infusion, decoction, tea, expressed juice.

Rupturewort *Herniara glabra.*
COMMON NAME: herniary, breastwort.
OCCURRENCE: found in temperate and southern Europe and Russian Asia. It is a British native plant, particularly in southern and central England.
PARTS USED: the herb, which contains the alkaloid paronychine, and a crystalline principle called herniarne.
MEDICINAL USES: astringent, diuretic. This is a very active drug

which has been successful in treating catarrhal infections of the bladder and oedema of cardiac or kidney origins.
ADMINISTERED AS: infusion.

Sabadilla *Veratrum sabadilla* or *Veratrum officinale.*
COMMON NAME: cevadilla, sabadillermer, caustic barley, *Schoenocaulon officinale, Melanthian sabadilla, Helonias officinalis, Sabadilla officinarum, Asagraea officinalis.*
OCCURRENCE: grows in southern North America, guatemala, Venezuela and Mexico.
PARTS USED: the seeds. They contain several alkaloids including veratrine, sabadillie, sabadine, sabadinine and cevadine, which hydrolyzes to cevine. They also contain voatric acid, cevadic acid, resin and fat.
MEDICINAL USES: drastic emetic and cathartic, vermifuge. The powdered seeds have been used to expel parasitic worms and to kill and remove parasitic mites or other vermin from the hair. An extract called veratria is derived from the seeds and despite it being highly poisonous, it is occasionally taken internally in minute doses. When taken internally, it can ease acute rheumatic pain and gout and also help some inflammatory diseases. Veratria is more commonly used as an ointment for neuralgia and rheumatism. This drug has a powerful action on the heart causing it to slow and eventually stop beating entirely.
ADMINISTERED AS: powdered seeds, ointment.

Saffron *Crocus sativus.*
COMMON NAME: crocus, karcom, Alicante saffron, Valencia saffron, krokos, gatinais, saffron, hay saffron, saffron crocus.
OCCURRENCE: grown from Persia and Kurdistan in the east to most European countries including Great Britain.
PARTS USED: the dried flower pistils. These parts contain an essen-

tial oil composed of terpenes, terepene alcohols and esters, a coloured glycoside called crocin and a bitter glucoside, called picrocrocin.
MEDICINAL USES: carminative, diaphoretic, emmenagogue. This herb is used as a diaphoretic drug for children and can also benefit female hysteria, absent or painful menstruation and stop chronic haemorrhage of the uterus in adults.
ADMINISTERED AS: tincture, powdered saffron.

Saffron, Meadow *Colchicum autumnale.*
COMMON NAME: colchicum, naked ladies.
OCCURRENCE: grows wild in North Africa and Europe and is found in meadows and limestone areas in the British Isles.
PARTS USED: the root and seeds.
MEDICINAL USES: cathartic, emetic, anti-rheumatic. This herb is very useful for acute rheumatic and gouty ailments, and it is normally taken along with an alkaline diuretic for best results. The active chemical in the plant is colchinine, an alkaline substance which is very poisonous. It has sedative effects and particularly acts on the bowels and kidneys. It acts as an irritant poison in large doses, and can cause undue depression. As such, care should be used when utilizing this herb.
ADMINISTERED AS: fluid extract, powdered root, tincture, solid extract.

Sage, Common *Salvia officinalis.*
COMMON NAME: garden sage, red sage, saurge, broad-leaved white sage, *Salvia salvatrix.*
OCCURRENCE: native to the northern Mediterranean and cultivated through Britain, France and Germany.
PARTS USED: the leaves, whole herb. The herb contains a volatile oil, tannin and resin and is distilled to produce sage oil. This is

made up of salvene, pinene, cineol, vorneol, thujone and some esters.
MEDICINAL USES: stimulant, astringent, tonic, carminative, aromatic. Sage makes an excellent gargle for relaxed throat and tonsils, bleeding gums, laryngitis and ulcerated throat. Sage tea is valuable against delirium of fevers, nervous excitement and accompanying brain and nervous diseases; as a stimulant tonic in stomach and nervous system complaints and in weak digestion. It also works as an emmenagogue, in treating typhoid fever, bilious and liver problems, kidney troubles and lung or stomach haemorrhages. The infusion is used in head colds, quinsy, measles, painful joints, lethargy, palsy and nervous headaches. Fresh leaves are rubbed on the teeth to cleanse them and strengthen gums—even today sage is included in toothpowders. The oil of sage was used to remove mucus collections from the respiratory organs and is included in embrocations for rheumatism. The herb is also applied warm as a poultice.
ADMINISTERED AS: infusion, essential oil, tea and poultice.

Salep: **early purple orchid**, *Orchis mascula*; **spotted orchid**, *Orchis maculata*; **marsh orchid**, *Orchis latifolia*.
COMMON NAME: saloop, schlep, satrion, Levant salep.
OCCURRENCE: *Orchis mascula* is found in woods throughout England. *O. maculata* grows wild on heaths and commons; *O. latifolia* is found growing in marshes and damp pastures across Great Britain.
PARTS USED: the tuberous root, which contains mucilage, sugar, starch and volatile oil.
MEDICINAL USES: very nutritive, demulcent. This herb is used as a food item for convalescent people and children, made with milk or water and flavoured. It is prepared in a similar way to arrowroot. A decoction with sugar, spice or wine was given to invalids

to build them up. The root is used to stop irritation of the gastro-intestinal canal and for invalids suffering from bilious fevers or chronic diarrhoea. In the old sailing ships, salep was carried and used as an emergency food source. It was sold on street corners in London as a hot drink, before COFFEE replaced its use as a beverage.
ADMINISTERED AS: decoction, dietary item.

Samphire *Crithmum maritimum.*
COMMON NAME: sea fennel, crest marine, sampier, rock fennel, rock samphire.
OCCURRENCE: found on rocks or salt marshes around the west or south of England but rare in the North and Scotland.
PARTS USED: the herb.
MEDICINAL USES: an infusion of samphire has a diuretic effect and acts on the kidneys. It is reputed to be an excellent treatment for obesity. It is eaten as a condiment, as a salad ingredient or pickled.
ADMINISTERED AS: infusion.

Sandalwood *Santalum album.*
COMMON NAME: santalwood, sanders-wood.
OCCURRENCE: a tree native to India and the Malay Archipelago.
PARTS USED: the wood oil.
MEDICINAL USES: aromatic, antiseptic, diuretic. The oil is given internally for chronic mucous conditions, e.g. bronchitis, inflammation of the bladder. It is also used in chronic cystitis, gleet and gonorrhoea. The oil is used in aromatherapy to lessen tension and anxiety and it was also considered a sexual stimulant in folk traditions. The fluid extract of sandalwood may be better tolerated by some people than the oil.
ADMINISTERED AS: wood oil, fluid extract.

Sarsaparilla, Jamaica *Smilax ornata.*
COMMON NAME: red-bearded sarsaparilla, *Smilax medica, Smilax officinalis.*
OCCURRENCE: a perennial climbing plant which grows in central America, primarily Costa Rica. It is termed Jamaican sarsaparilla as the plant was exported to Europe through Jamaica.
PARTS USED: the root, which is composed of starch, sarsapic acid, the glucoside sarsaponin and palmitic, stearic, behenic, oleic and linoleic fatty acids. The active principle is a crystalline compound called porillin or smilacin.
MEDICINAL USES: alterative, tonic, diaphoretic, diuretic. This root was introduced into Europe in 1563 as a remedy for syphilis. It is used in other chronic diseases, particularly rheumatism or skin diseases. It is still considered an excellent blood purifier, often given in conjunction with SASSAFRAS or BURDOCK. When smoked, Jamaican sarsaparilla was recommended for asthma.
ADMINISTERED AS: powdered root, fluid extract, solid extract.

Sassafras *Sassafras officinale.*
COMMON NAME: laurus sassafras, sassafrax, *Sassafras radix, Sassafras varifolium.*
OCCURRENCE: native to the eastern United States and Canada then south to Mexico.
PARTS USED: the root-bark, root and pith. The root-bark contains a heavy and light volatile oil, resin, wax, tannic acid, lignin, starch and camphorous matter. The pith is made up of mucilage which is used as a demulcent. The bark yields an oil, which is mainly safrol. This is a heavy volatile oil associated with sassafras camphor when cold.
MEDICINAL USES: aromatic, stimulant, diaphoretic, alterative, diuretic. This herb is usually given in combination with other herbs, e.g. SARSAPARILLA, to treat chronic rheumatism, skin diseases or

syphilis. The oil relieves pain after childbirth and due to obstructed menstruation and also benefits gonorrhoea and gleet. A decoction of the pith is used as an eye wash in eye complaints and in general inflammations. Safrol, when taken internally, can produce narcotic poisoning, but when used externally it can be used for rheumatic pains and as a dental disinfectant.
ADMINISTERED AS: oil of sassafras, fluid extract, decoction.

Sassy bark *Erythrophloeum guineense.*
COMMON NAME: maneona bark, casca bark, doom bark, ordeal bark, saucy bark, red water bark, nkasa, *Cortex erythrophei.*
OCCURRENCE: a large tree native to the west coast of Africa in Upper Guinea, Senegal, Gambia and Sudan.
PARTS USED: the bark, which contains the poisonous chemical erythrophleine, tannin and resin.
MEDICINAL USES: narcotic, astringent, anodyne, laxative. It has been used successfully in dysentery, diarrhoea and passive haemorrhages. The chemical erythrophleine acts on the pulse rate, peristalsis and the nerve centres to cause relief from pain, purging and vomiting. It needs more research to see if erythrophleine would make a good anaesthetic drug. Since it is very poisonous and has severe effects on the body, it is rarely used in modern herbal medicine. In native West African cultures, this drug is given as an ordeal in trials of witchcraft and sorcery to determine the truth.
ADMINISTERED AS: fluid extract, powdered bark.

Savory, Summer *Satureja hortensis.*
COMMON NAME: garden savory.
OCCURRENCE: a shrub native to the Mediterranean region and introduced into Great Britain.
PARTS USED: the herb.

MEDICINAL USES: aromatic, carminative. This herb is mainly used in cookery, as a pot-herb or flavouring. In medicine, it is added to remedies to flavour and add warmth. It was formerly used for colic, flatulence and was considered a good expectorant. A sprig of summer savory rubbed on a wasp or bee sting relieves the pain quickly.
ADMINISTERED AS: fresh or dried herb.

Savine *Juniperus sabina.*
COMMON NAME: savin, savine tops.
OCCURRENCE: indigenous to the northern states in the USA and middle and southern Europe, e.g. Switzerland, Italy and Austria.
PARTS USED: the tops of the herb. It contains gallic acid, resin, chlorophyll, a volatile oil, lilgnin, calcium salts, gum and a fixed oil.
MEDICINAL USES: emmenagogue, diuretic, anthelmintic. This herb is rarely given internally as it is an irritant herb and also poisonous, whose use can be fatal if not properly managed. It is a powerful emmenagogue which can induce abortion when given in large doses—should never be taken when pregnant. It used to be administered with TANSY, PENNY ROYAL and HEMLOCK. As a vermifuge, it has been used for worms along with PINK ROOT and SENNA. Mainly used externally as an ointment for skin eruptions, blisters and syphilitic warts. It is said to remove warts from the hands.
ADMINISTERED AS: powdered herb, tincture, fluid extract.

Saw palmetto *Sarenoa serrulata.*
COMMON NAME: sabal, *Sabal serrulata.*
OCCURRENCE: native to the North Atlantic coast of the United States and southern California.
PARTS USED: the ripe fruit, which contains volatile oil, glucose and a fixed oil.

MEDICINAL USES: nutritive, tonic, diuretic, sedative. This herb affects the mucous membranes of the respiratory system to ease many diseases linked to chronic catarrh. Saw palmetto is a tissue-building herb which aids atony of the testicles or breasts. It reduces catarrhal irritation in the body and can ease catarrh of the bladder and urethra.
ADMINISTERED AS: solid extract, powdered fruit, fluid extract.

Saxifrage, Burnet *Pimpinella saxifraga.*
COMMON NAME: lesser burnet, saxifrage.
OCCURRENCE: found on dry, chalky pastures throughout the British Isles.
PARTS USED: the root and the herb.
MEDICINAL USES: resolvent, diaphoretic, diuretic, stomachic, aromatic, carminative. This herb is prescribed for flatulent indigestion, toothache, paralysis of the tongue, asthma and dropsy. A decoction is used as a gargle in throat infections and hoarseness. The herb was added to casks of beer or wine to impart its aromatic flavour to the drink.
ADMINISTERED AS: fresh root, decoction dried root.

Scullcap, Virginian *Scutellaria lateriflora.*
COMMON NAME: mad-dog scullcap, helmet flower, madweed, mad-dog weed, skullcap, Quaker bonnet.
OCCURRENCE: native to the United States of America.
PARTS USED: the herb, which contains a volatile oil called scutellonin, flavonoid glucosides including scutellonin and scutellanein, some bitter principle, sugar, cellulose, tannin and fat.
MEDICINAL USES: strong tonic, nervine, antispasmodic, astringent. This herb is an invaluable tonic for the nervous system treating nervous headaches, anxiety, depression, insomnia and neuralgia. It is most beneficial in hysteria, convulsions, rickets, epilepsy

and Speakman's chorea where it soothes nervous excitement and induces sleep without any unpleasant side effects. The bitter taste of the herb stimulates and strengthens the digestion. It is said that many cases of hydrophobia have been cured by the use of this herb alone. The European species, *Scutellaria galericulata*, was once used for malaria and it shares the nervine qualities of Virginian scullcap. This herb may be difficult to obtain as most commercial supplies of it are adulterated with wood sage (*Teucrium scorodonia*).
ADMINISTERED AS: fluid extract, infusion, decoction, powdered herb.

Scurvy grass *Cochlearia officinalis*.
COMMON NAME: spoonwort.
OCCURRENCE: native to the coastline of Scotland, Ireland and England; also found in the sea coasts of northern and western Europe, the Arctic Circle and at altitude on the mountain chains of Europe.
PARTS USED: the herb.
MEDICINAL USES: stimulant, aperient, diuretic, antiscorbutic. It was formerly used on sea voyages to prevent scurvy. The essential oil from the herb is beneficial in cases of rheumatism or paralysis. When made into scurvy grass ale it was drunk as a tonic.
ADMINISTERED AS: infusion, essential oil.

Self-heal *Prunella vulgaris*.
COMMON NAME: prunella, all-heal, hook-heal, slough-heal, brunella, heart of the Earth, blue curls, siclewort.
OCCURRENCE: a very abundant wild plant in woods and fields all over Europe and Great Britain.
PARTS USED: the whole herb, containing a volatile oil, a bitter principle, tannin, sugar and cellulose.

MEDICINAL USES: astringent, styptic and tonic. An infusion of the herb is taken internally for sore throats, internal bleeding, leucorrhoea and as a general strengthener.
ADMINISTERED AS: infusion, injection and decoction.

Senega *Polygala senega.*
COMMON NAME: snake root, seneca, milkwort, mountain flax, rattlesnake root, senega snakeroot, seneka, *Senegae radix*, *Polygala virginiana*, *Plantula marilandica*, *Senega officinalis.*
OCCURRENCE: grows wild throughout central and western North America.
PARTS USED: the dried root, which contains polygalic acid, virgineic acid, pectic and tannic acids, fixed oil, albumen, sugar and various mineral salts. The active chemical is called senegin which is almost identical to the saponin chemical found in SOAPWORT (*Saponaria officinale*).
MEDICINAL USES: stimulant, expectorant, diaphoretic, diuretic, emmenagogue. It is highly effective in treating acute bronchial catarrh, chronic pneumonia or bronchitis and kidney-related dropsy. senega is also of benefit for croup, whooping cough and rheumatism. The ancient herbalists of Greek or Roman times considered senega of identical action with IPECACUANHA (*Cephaelis ipecacuanha*). In large doses senega is an emetic and cathartic drug, and overdoses are possible.
ADMINISTERED AS: powder, fluid extract, syrup, tincture, infusion.

Senna, Alexandrian *Cassia acutifolia*; **Senna, East Indian** *Cassia angustifolia.*
COMMON NAME: Nubian senna, Egyptian senna, tinnevelly senna, *Cassia senna*, *Cassia lenitiva*, *Cassia lanceolata*, *Cassia officinalis*, *Cassia aethiopica*, *Senna acutifolia.*
OCCURRENCE: *C. acutifolia* is native to the upper and middle Nile

in Egypt and Sudan. *C. angustifolia* is indigenous to southern Arabia and is cultivated in southern and eastern India.
PARTS USED: the dried leaflets and pods. The active principles of senna can be extracted using water or dilute alcohol. The drug contains anthraquinone derivatives and their glucosides, as well as cathartic acid as its active chemicals.
MEDICINAL USES: laxative, purgative, cathartic. This drug acts primarily on the lower bowel, acts locally upon the intestinal wall, increasing the peristaltic movements of the colon. The taste is nauseating and prone to cause sickness and griping pains. It is generally combined with aromatics, e.g. GINGER or CINNAMON and stimulants to modify senna's deleterious effects. When the problems are overcome, senna is a very good medicine for children, delicate women and elderly persons. Senna pods have milder effects than the leaves and lack their griping effects.
ADMINISTERED AS: infusion, powdered leaves, syrup, fluid extract, tincture, dried pods.

Sheep's sorrel *Rumex acetosella.*
COMMON NAME: field sorrel.
OCCURRENCE: this grows in pastures and dry places around the globe, except in the tropics and is abundant in the British Isles.
PARTS USED: the herb.
MEDICINAL USES: diaphoretic, diuretic, refrigerant. The fresh juice of the herb is used for kidney and urinary diseases. Less active than SORREL (*Rumex acetosa*).
ADMINISTERED AS: expressed juice.

Shepherd's purse *Capsella bursa-pastoris.*
COMMON NAME: shepherd's bag, shepherd's scrip, lady's purse, witches' pouches, case-weed, pick-pocket, blindweed, pepper and

salt, sanguinary, mother's heart, poor man's parmacettie, clappedepouch.

OCCURRENCE: native to Europe and found all over the world outside tropical zones.

PARTS USED: the whole plant which contains various chemicals which have not yet been entirely analyzed but they include an organic acid, a volatile oil, a fixed oil, a tannate, an alkaloid and a resin.

MEDICINAL USES: haemostatic, antiscorbutic, diuretic, stimulant. As an infusion of the dried plant, shepherd's purse is one of the best specifics for arresting bleeding of all kinds, particularly from the kidneys, uterus, stomach or lungs. It is said to be as effective as ERGOT or GOLDEN SEAL. It has been used for diarrhoea, haemorrhoids, dysentery, dropsy and kidney complaints. Shepherd's purse is an important remedy in catarrhal infections of the bladder and ureter and in ulcerated and abscess of the bladder where it increases the flow of urine and provides relief. Externally, the bruised herb is used as a poultice on bruised and strained areas, rheumatic joints and some skin problems. Since the herb tastes slightly unpleasant it is normally taken internally with other herbs to disguise the flavour, e.g. COUCH GRASS, JUNIPER, PELLITORY-OF-THE-WALL.

ADMINISTERED AS: fluid extract, poultice, decoction, infusion.

Silverweed *Potentilla anserina.*

COMMON NAME: trailing tansy, wild tansy, goosewort, silvery cinquefoil, goose grey, goose tansy, wild agrimony, moor grass, prince's feathers.

OCCURRENCE: very abundant in Great Britain and across temperate regions from Lapland to the Azores. It also grows in New Zealand, Chile, Armenia and China.

PARTS USED: the herb, which contains tannin.

MEDICINAL USES: astringent, tonic. An infusion is used as a lotion for bleeding haemorrhoids, as a gargle for sore throats and for cramps in the abdomen, stomach or heart. The infusion may also be used as a compress. A tea of Silverweed has been good for tetanus infections, for malarial infections, in gravel and as a specific in jaundice. A decoction of silverweed is useful for mouth ulcers, spongy gums, fixing loose teeth, toothache and preserving gums from scurvy. A distilled water made from the herb was used as a cosmetic to remove freckles, spots and pimples and to reduce the skin damage after sunburn.
ADMINISTERED AS: decoction, infusion, poultice, distilled water.

Simaruba *Simaruba amara.*
COMMON NAME: dysentery bark, mountain damson, slave wood, maruba, sumaruppa, bitter damson, quassia simaruba.
OCCURRENCE: native to French Guiana, Brazil, Florida and the islands of Dominica, Martinique, St. Lucia, St. Vincent and Barbados.
PARTS USED: the bark, which contains a volatile oil, malic and gallic acids, lignin, resinous matter, various mineral salts and a bitter principle very similar to quassin.
MEDICINAL USES: bitter tonic. It was used successfully against dysentery in France from 1718 onwards. The drug restores lost tone of the intestines and encourages the patient to sleep. It is also useful in loss of appetite, weakened digestion and when convalescing after a fever. In large doses, simaruba can cause sickness and vomiting, so care should be taken when using this drug. It is seldom used in herbal medicine today.
ADMINISTERED AS: infusion, fluid extract.

Skunk cabbage *Symplocarpus foetidus.*
COMMON NAME: dracontium, skunkweed, meadow cabbage, pole-

cat weed, *Dracontium foetidum*, *Spathyema foetida*, *Ictodes foetidus*.
OCCURRENCE: grows in moist places across the middle and northern United States of America.
PARTS USED: the root, which contains resin, silica, iron, manganese, an acrid principle and a volatile oil.
MEDICINAL USES: antispasmodic, diaphoretic, expectorant, narcotic, sedative. This plant is so-named as it has an unpleasant odour when bruised. The root has been used for asthma, chronic rheumatism, chorea, dropsy, hysteria and chronic catarrh. It is good for tightness of the chest, irritant coughs and other spasmodic respiratory disorders. The herb is also believed to be effective against epilepsy and convulsions which can occur during pregnancy or labour. It has a diuretic action and can be used to calm the nervous system. Skunk-cabbage forms an ingredient in well-known herbal ointments and powders.
ADMINISTERED AS: powdered root, tincture, fluid extract.

Slippery elm *Ulmus fulva*.
COMMON NAME: red elm, moose elm, Indian elm.
OCCURRENCE: the United States and Canada.
PARTS USED: the inner bark of the tree, which contains mucilage similar to that of flax, starch and calcium oxalate.
MEDICINAL USES: demulcent, emollient, expectorant, diuretic, nutritive, pectoral. This is one of the most valuable remedies in herbal practice. Finely powdered bark makes very good gruel or food which can be used in all cases of weakness, stomach inflammation, bronchitis, etc. It has a soothing and healing action on all the parts it comes into contact with. A drink of the powder and water called Slippery elm food is excellent in cases of irritation of the mucous membrane of the stomach and intestines, induces sleep and gives very good results in gastritis, colitis and enteritis and

gastric catarrh. May also be employed as a heart and lung remedy and is used in typhoid fever.

The coarse powdered bark is the finest available poultice for all inflamed areas, ulcers, wounds, burns, boils, skin diseases, etc. It is utilized by various methods in treating many disorders of the bowel and urinary systems. It is also used to remove worms and is an ingredient in many specialist preparations, e.g. poultices, ointments, etc.

ADMINISTERED AS: infusion, injection, poultice, ointment and dietary item.

Smartweed *Polygonum hydropiper.*

COMMON NAME: water pepper, pepper plant, smartass, ciderage, red knees, culrage, biting persicaria, bloodwort, arsesmart.

OCCURRENCE: a native plant of most parts of Europe and Russian Asia up to the Arctic regions. Also seen in Great Britain and Ireland, although rarer in Scotland. It mainly grows in areas that are under water in the winter period.

PARTS USED: the whole herb and the leaves. The active principle is called polygonic acid but its action is not fully understood. It is destroyed by heat or drying.

MEDICINAL USES: stimulant, diuretic, diaphoretic, emmenagogue. As a cold water infusion, this herb is used for amenorrhoea, gravel, coughs and colds and gout. It is also of benefit in dysentery, sore mouths, bowel complaints, jaundice and dropsy. After simmering with water and vinegar, the herb has been utilized on gangrenous or dead tissue, applied to chronic ulcers and haemorrhoidal tumours. In poultice form, smartweed has been used in chronic erysipelas infections, flatulent colic, cholera and rheumatism. There is a tradition which is mentioned in old herbals, that if a handful of the plant is placed under the saddle of a horse then it will be able to travel for some time be-

fore requiring feeding or watering. This belief dates back to the Ancient Greek period.
ADMINISTERED AS: infusion, tincture, fluid extract.

Snapdragon *Antirrhinum magus.*
COMMON NAME: calves, snout, lyons snap.
OCCURRENCE: naturalized in Great Britain and is a garden plant.
PARTS USED: the leaves.
MEDICINAL USES: bitter, stimulant. The fresh leaves have been applied as a poultice to tumours and ulcers. In old herbals, it is mentioned that the herb protects against witchcraft and that it makes the wearer "look gracious in the sight of people."
ADMINISTERED AS: poultice.

Soap tree *Quillaja saponia.*
COMMON NAME: quillaia, soap bark, cullay, Panama bark.
OCCURRENCE: native to Chile and Peru in South America.
PARTS USED: the dried inner bark, which contains calcium exalate, can sugar and saponin which is made from a mixture of two glucosides—guillaic acid and guillaia—sapotoxin. The active principles are the same as those found in SENEGA.
MEDICINAL USES: alterative, expectorant, detergent, diuretic, stimulating, sternutatory. This bark can be used in aortic hypertrophy. Since Saponin is a powerful irritant and muscular poison, it can be fatal if used in too large doses and is only occasionally used today. The bark has been used to produce a foam head on beverages and for washing clothes and hair.
ADMINISTERED AS: injection, tincture, powdered bark.

Soapwort *Saponaria officinalis.*
COMMON NAME: latherwort, soaproot, bruisewort, fuller's herb, crow soap, sweet betty, wild sweet william, bouncing bet.

OCCURRENCE: a common garden plant in Great Britain and it also grows wild in central and southern Europe.
PARTS USED: the dried root and leaves. The root contains gum, resin, woody fibre, mucilage and saponin.
MEDICINAL USES: alterative, detergent, tonic, sternutatory. This herb has been used for scrofula and other skin complaints and in jaundice and other visceral obstructions. It is also good for chronic venereal diseases and in rheumatism or skin eruptions due to infection with syphilis. This drug should be very carefully administered due to the very poisonous nature of saponin. In large doses, soapwort is strongly purgative so should only be given by a qualified herbalist. Soapwort is also used to clean clothes, skin and hair and is an ingredient of most herbal shampoo.
ADMINISTERED AS: decoction, expressed juice from fresh root, fluid extract.

Solomon's seal *Polygonatum multiflorum.*
COMMON NAME: lady's seals, St. Mary's seal, sigillum sanctae Mariae.
OCCURRENCE: a native plant of northern Europe and Siberia. It is found wild in some localities in England but naturalized in Scotland and Ireland.
PARTS USED: the rhizome which contains asparagin, gum, sugar, starch, pectin and convallarin, one of the active chemicals in LILY OF THE VALLEY.
MEDICINAL USES: astringent,

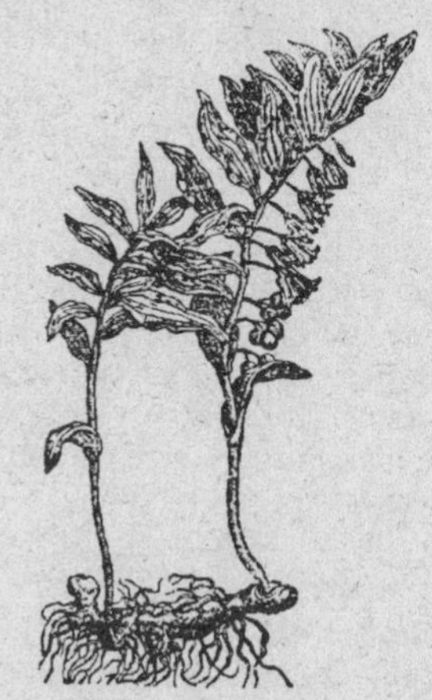
Solomon's seal

demulcent, tonic. When combined with other herbs, it is good for bleeding of the lungs and pulmonary complaints. It is used on its own in female complaints and as a poultice for tumours, inflammations, bruises and haemorrhoids. As it is mucilaginous, it makes a very good healing and restorative tonic for inflammation of the bowels and stomach, haemorrhoids and chronic dysentery. A decoction was used to cure erysipelas and was taken by people with broken bones, as Solomon's Seal was supposed to 'encourage the bones to knit'. A distilled water prepared from the root was used as a cosmetic to remove spots, freckles and marks from the skin.
ADMINISTERED AS: decoction, infusion, poultice, distilled water.

Sorrel *Rumex acetosa.*
COMMON NAME: garden sorrel, green sauce, sour grabs, sour suds, cuckoo sorrow, cuckoo's meate, gowke-meat.
OCCURRENCE: indigenous to Britain and found in moist meadows throughout Europe.
PARTS USED: the leaves, dried and fresh.
MEDICINAL USES: refrigerant, diuretic, antiscorbutic. Sorrel is given as a cooling drink in all febrile conditions and can help correct scrofulous deposits. Its astringent qualities meant it was formerly used to stop haemorrhages and was applied as a poultice on cutaneous tumours. Sorrel juice and vinegar are said to cure ringworm, while a decoction was made to cure jaundice, ulcerated bowel, and gravel and stone in the kidneys.
ADMINISTERED AS: expressed juice, decoction, poultice and dried leaves.

Spearmint *Mentha viridis.*
COMMON NAME: mackerel mint, Our Lady's mint, green mint, spire mint, sage of Bethlehem, fish mint, lamb mint, menthe de Notre

Dame, erba Santa Maria, *Mentha spicata*, *Mentha crispa*, yerba buena.
OCCURRENCE: originally a Mediterranean native and was introduced into the British Isles by the Romans.
PARTS USED: the herb and essential oil. The main component of the essential oil is carvone along with phellandrine, limonene and dihydrocarveol acetate. The oil also has the esters of acetic, butyric and caproic acids within it.
MEDICINAL USES: antispasmodic, aromatic, carminative, stimulant. This herb is very similar to peppermint, but it seems to be less powerful. It is more suited to children's remedies. A distilled water from spearmint is used to relieve hiccoughs, flatulence and indigestion while the infusion is good for fevers, inflammatory diseases and all infantile troubles. Spearmint is considered a specific in stopping nausea and vomiting and in easing the pain due to colic. As a homoeopathic remedy, spearmint has been used for strangury, gravel and as a local application for painful haemorrhoids.
ADMINISTERED AS: distilled water, infusion, tincture, fluid extract.

Spearwort, Lesser *Ranunculus flammula*.
OCCURRENCE: a very common plant throughout Britain, growing in wet and boggy heaths and commons.
PARTS USED: the whole plant.
MEDICINAL USES: rubefacient, emetic. The bruised leaves have a long history of use on the Isle of Skye and in the Highlands of Scotland in raising blisters. A distilled water from the plant is used as a painless emetic drug while a tincture is good at curing ulcers.
ADMINISTERED AS: distilled water, tincture, poultice.

Speedwell, Common *Veronica officinalis*.
COMMON NAME: bird's-eye, cat's-eye.

Occurrence: a common wild plant in Europe and Great Britain.
Parts used: the herb.
Medicinal uses: diaphoretic, alterative, expectorant, astringent, diuretic, tonic. Lesser spearwort was formerly used in pectoral and nephritic complaints, haemorrhages, skin diseases and in treating wounds. An infusion of the dried herb is good for catarrh, coughs and most skin problems. May promote menstruation.
Administered as: infusion and dried herb.

Sphagnum moss *Sphagnum cymbifolium.*
Common name: bog moss.
Occurrence: found in wet and boggy land, normally on peat soils on mountains and moors in Scotland, England, Ireland and parts of western Europe.
Parts used: the moss, which is made up of plant cells which are penetrated with a system of tubes and air spaces. This capillary tube system makes the moss resemble a very fine sponge and allows the plant to absorb huge quantities of water.
Medicinal uses: wound dressing. The use of sphagnum as a dressing for wounds can be dated back to the Battle of Flodden. There is a long history of use in Lapland where the dried moss is used as a mattress and blankets for infants. The moss has many advantages over other surgical dressings, e.g. cotton wool. Prepared moss can retain twice as much moisture as cotton; a 2oz dressing can absorb up to 2lb of liquid. This means that dressings need to be changed less frequently with less disturbance to the patient. In many times of war sphagnum was prepared in gauze bags, often in association with garlic for its antiseptic qualities. Sphagnum moss also has an antibiotic action due to micro-organisms associated with the plant which aids healing. The moss has also been used as bedding in stables and for hanging baskets and other gardening applications.

Spinach *Spinacio oleracea.*
OCCURRENCE: originally native to Persia and Asia and was introduced into Europe in the fifteenth century.
PARTS USED: the leaves, which contain iron, nitrogenous substances, hydrocarbons, chlorophyll and vitamins A and D.
MEDICINAL USES: nutritive, antiscorbutic. Spinach is primarily used as a food source as it is a good source of iron and vitamins. Experiments have shown the benefit of eating spinach on people weakened by illness.
ADMINISTERED AS: expressed juice, dietary item.

Spindle tree *Euonymus atropurpureus. Euonymus europoeus.*
COMMON NAME: Indian arrowroot, burning bush, wahoo, gatten, pigwood, dogwood, skewerwood, prickwood, gadrose, fusanum, fusoria.
OCCURRENCE: *Euonymus europoeus* is found in copses and hedges across Great Britain. *E. atropurpureus* is commonly found in the eastern United States and is the variety normally used in herbal medicine.
PARTS USED: the root, bark and berries. The chief constituents of the plant include an intensely bitter principle called euonymin resin, euonic acid, asparagin, resins, fat, dulcitol and a crystalline glucoside.
MEDICINAL USES: alterative, cholagogue, laxative, hepatic stimulant, tonic. This drug is particularly good in liver complaints which follow or accompany fever, and in stimulating the liver and producing a free flow of bile. Depending on the dose given euonymin has different effects on the digestive system. In large doses it irritates the intestine and has cathartic effects, but in smaller doses it can stimulate the appetite and the flow of gastric juices. The herb is normally administered with other tonic or laxative herbs for best results.

ADMINISTERED AS: pills, powdered root or bark, decoction, fluid extract.

St John's wort *Hypericum perforatum.*
OCCURRENCE: found in woods, hedges, roadsides and meadows across Britain, Europe and Asia.
PARTS USED: the herb and flowers.
MEDICINAL USES: aromatic, astringent, resolvent, expectorant, diuretic and nervine. It is generally utilized in all pulmonary complaints, bladder trouble, suppression of urine, dysentery, diarrhoea and jaundice. It is good against hysteria, nervous depression, haemorrhages, coughing up blood and dispelling worms from the body. If children have a problem with night incontinence, an infusion of St John's wort taken before bed will stop the problem. The herb is used externally to break up hard tissues, e.g. tumours, bruising and swollen, hard breasts when feeding infants.
ADMINISTERED AS: an infusion and poultice.

Stavesacre *Delphinium staphisagria.*
COMMON NAME: starvesacre, staphisagris, lousewort.
OCCURRENCE: indigenous to southern Europe and Asia Minor, and is now cultivated in France and Italy.
PARTS USED: the dried ripe seeds. The main components of the seeds are alkaloid compounds including the poisonous delphinine, delphisine, delphinoidine, staphisagroine and staphisagrine, which may make up twenty five per cent of the seeds.
MEDICINAL USES: vermifuge, vermin-destroying, violent emetic and cathartic. The seeds are so very poisonous that they are rarely taken internally. Occasionally, the powdered seeds may be used as a purge in treating dropsy, with the dose monitored very carefully. The seeds are used externally as a parasiticide to kill lice of

the genus *Pediculus*, and as a poultice or decoction compress on some skin eruptions and scrofula. The extracted alkaloid delphinine has been used both internally and externally to ease neuralgia. It resembles ACONITE in its action, slowing the pulse and respiration rates, paralysing the spinal cord and leading to death by asphyxia when taken in large doses. It can be used as an antidote to poisoning by strychnine.
ADMINISTERED AS: ointment, expressed oil, powdered seeds, decoction, poultice, fluid extract.

Stockholm tar *Pinus sylvestris* (and other species).
COMMON NAME: tar, *Pix liquida*.
OCCURRENCE: obtained from various *Pinus* species grown across the northern hemisphere in Sweden, Russia, North America and Switzerland.
PARTS USED: the tar is an impure turpentine obtained from the stems and roots of *Pinus* species by destructive distillation.
MEDICINAL USES: antiseptic, diuretic, diaphoretic, expectorant, stimulant. It may be used for chronic coughs and consumption but is mainly used externally as a cutaneous stimulant and as an ointment for eczema. It is mainly used in veterinary practices.
ADMINISTERED AS: ointment, fluid extract.

Stramonium *Datura stramonium*.
COMMON NAME: thornapple, jimsonweed, Jamestownweed, devil's apple, devil's trumpet, datura, mad apple, stinkweed, apple of Peru.
OCCURRENCE: a plant of unknown origin that is currently found throughout the world except in cold or Arctic areas.
PARTS USED: the whole plant has medicinal qualities but it is the leaves and seeds that are most commonly used today. The leaves contain the same alkaloids as BELLADONNA, but in slightly smaller amounts. The alkaloids include lyoscyamine, atropine, lyoscine along

with malic acid, volatile oil, gum, resin and starch. The seeds are made up of fixed oil and the same alkaloids as the leaves, but the fixed oil makes the alkaloids difficult to extract so the leaves are the most extensively utilized.

MEDICINAL USES: antispasmodic, anodyne, narcotic. A herb which acts in a very similar manner to belladonna except it does not cause constipation. An extract of the seeds is given in pill form to stop coughing in spasmodic bronchial asthma, to ease whooping cough and spasm of the bladder. It is considered a better cough remedy than opium, but is used with extreme care as it can act as a narcotic poison in overdoses. When smoked with tobacco, alone or with other herbs, e.g. SAGE and BELLADONNA, stramonium can ease asthma by relaxing spasms of the bronchioles during an attack. Taken in this form, it can also help control the spasms that occur in Parkinson's disease. The herb can relieve the pain of sciatica and rheumatism when used externally in the form of an ointment.. Signs of an overdose of stramonium include dryness of the throat and mouth and an overdose can cause double vision, thirst, palpitations, restlessness, confusion and hallucinations. This drug is highly toxic and should only be used under the guidance of a herbal medicine practitioner or doctor. In India, thieves and assassins used to give their victims Stramonium in order to make them insensible while history states that the herb was taken by the priests of Apollo at Delphi, in Ancient Greece, to assist them in their prophecies.

Stramonium was considered to be a plant which aided witches in their ill-doing, and during the time of the witch and wizard hunt in England, it was exceedingly dangerous to grow stramonium in your garden as it was said to confirm the supernatural powers of the householder. Many people were sentenced to death purely because stramonium was found in their garden.

ADMINISTERED AS: powdered leaves, powdered seeds, fluid extract, tincture and ointment.

Strawberry *Fragaria vesca.*
OCCURRENCE: found through the whole of the northern hemisphere, excluding the tropics.
PARTS USED: the leaves, which contain cissotanic, malic and citric acids, sugar, mucilage and a volatile aromatic chemical which is, as yet, unidentified.
MEDICINAL USES: laxative, diuretic, astringent. The berries are of great benefit for rheumatic gout while the root is good against diarrhoea. The leaves have similar properties and are used to stop dysentery. Fresh strawberries remove discolouration of the teeth if the juice is left on for about five minutes and then the teeth are cleaned with warm water, to which a pinch of bicarbonate of soda has been added. Sunburn could be relieved by rubbing a cut strawberry over a freshly washed face.
ADMINISTERED AS: infusion, fresh berries.

Strophanthus *Strophanthus kombé.*
COMMON NAME: kombe seeds, *Strophanthus hispidus*, *S. semina.*
OCCURRENCE: native to tropical East Africa.
PARTS USED: the seeds. These contain the glucoside strophanthus, the alkaloid inoeine and a fixed oil.
MEDICINAL USES: cardiac tonic. This drug has a large influence on the circulatory system. It is used in chronic heart weakness, muscular debility of the heart and in cardiac pains with difficult or laboured breathing. It acts in the same way as digitalis (FOXGLOVE, *Digitalis purpurea*), but with increased digestive disturbance and strophanthus does not have a cumulative poisoning effect. Strophanthus has diuretic powers and is beneficial in dropsy, particularly when related to heart problems. In urgent cases, the intra-

venous injection of strophanthus can be used to increase circulation. The strength and power of the seeds are highly variable, and the seeds are so highly poisonous that they should only be used under medical supervision. In Africa, strophanthus is used as an arrow poison.
ADMINISTERED AS: liquid extract, tincture, solid extract.

Sumbul *Ferula sumbul.*
COMMON NAME: musk root, ouchi, ofnokgi, racine de sumbul, sumbulwurzel, moschuswurzel, jatamarsi, *Sumbul radix.*
OCCURRENCE: thought to be native to Turkestan, northern India and Russia.
PARTS USED: the root and rhizome. They contain two balsamic resins (thought to cause the strong musk-like odour), wax, gum, a bitter substance, a volatile oil, starch and angelic and valeric acids.
MEDICINAL USES: nerve stimulant, antispasmodic, tonic. Sumbul resembles VALERIAN in action and is very good for various hysterical conditions. It is thought to have a specific action on the pelvic organs and is used for dysmenorrhoea and similar female problems. Sumbul acts as a stimulant of the mucous membranes easing chronic diarrhoea and dysentery as well as pneumonia, chronic bronchitis and asthma. The side effects of the drug can occur producing narcotic symptoms, confusion, tingling feelings and a strong odour on the breath which may take two days to disappear.
ADMINISTERED AS: solid extract, tincture, fluid extract.

Sundew *Drosera rotundifolia.*
COMMON NAME: roundleaved sundew, dew plant, red rot, youthwort, rosa solis, herba rosellae, rosée du soleil.
OCCURRENCE: an insectivorous plant found in bogs, wet places and river edges throughout Britain, Europe, India, China, North and South America and Russian Asia.

PARTS USED: the air-dried flowering plant.
MEDICINAL USES: pectoral, expectorant, demulcent, anti-asthmatic. In small doses sundew is a specific in dry, spasmodic, tickling coughs and is considered very good in whooping cough, for which it may also be used as a prophylactic drug. The fresh juice is used to remove corns and warts. In America, the sundew has been advocated as a cure for old age and has been used with colloidal silicates in cases of thickening of arteries due to old age, or calcium or fat deposition.
ADMINISTERED AS: fluid extract, expressed juice, solid extract.

Sunflower *Helicanthus annuus*.
COMMON NAME: helianthus, marigold of Peru, *Sola indianus*, *Chrysanthemum peruvianum*, *Corona solis*.
OCCURRENCE: native to Peru and Mexico and was introduced into America, Europe and Great Britain as a garden plant.
PARTS USED: the seeds. These contain a vegetable oil, carbonate of potash, tannin and vitamins B1, B3 and B6. The oil is expressed from the crushed seeds and, according to the range of temperature to which the seeds are heated, several grades of oil are obtained.
MEDICINAL USES: diuretic, expectorant. It has been used successfully in treating pulmonary, bronchial and laryngeal afflictions as

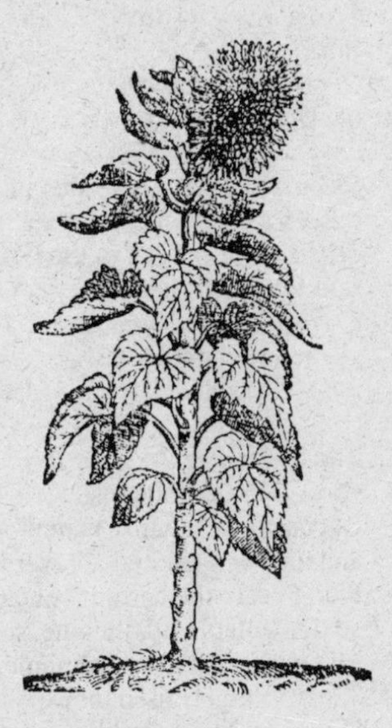

sunflower

well as whooping cough, colds and coughs. The leaves are used, in some parts of the world, to treat malaria and the tincture may replace quinine in easing intermittent fevers and the ague. Sunflowers produce the seed cake which is used as cattle food; the fresh leaves are given to poultry; the plants can be used as a vegetable; the stems are used as bedding for ducks; the plant used for silage, fuel, manure, textiles and as a soil improver.
ADMINISTERED AS: sunflower oil, tincture, decoction, poultice.

Tag alder *Alnus semulata.*
COMMON NAME: smooth alder, red alder, common alder, *Alnus rubra.*
OCCURRENCE: a common tree found in Europe, Great Britain and the United States of America.
PARTS USED: the bark and cones.
MEDICINAL USES: tonic, alterative, emetic, astringent. This plant is good for scrofula, diarrhoea, dyspepsia, indigestion, secondary syphilis and debility of the stomach. A decoction of the cones was said to be astringent in effect and of use in all types of haemorrhages. The bark was also of benefit to some cutaneous diseases and intermittent fevers.
ADMINISTERED AS: infusion, decoction, fluid extract.

Tansy *Tanacetum vulgare.*
COMMON NAME: buttons.
OCCURRENCE: a hardy perennial plant, commonly seen in hedges and on waste ground all over Europe and Great Britain.
PARTS USED: the herb. It contains the chemicals tanacetin, tannic acid, a volatile oil, thujone, sugar and a colouring matter.
MEDICINAL USES: anthelmintic, tonic, emmenagogue, stimulant. Tansy is largely used for expelling worms from children. It is good in female disorders, like hysteria and nausea and in kidney weak-

ness. The herb is also used for slight fevers, for allaying spasms and as a nervine drug. In large doses, the herb is violently irritant and induces venous congestion of the abdominal organs. In Scotland, an infusion was administered to cure gout. Tansy essential oil, when given in small doses, has helped in epilepsy and has also been used externally to help some eruptive diseases of the skin. Bruised fresh leaves can reduce swelling and relieve sprains, as can a hot infusion used as a poultice.
ADMINISTERED AS: essential oil, infusion, poultice, fresh leaves, solid extract.

Tarragon *Artemisia dracunculus.*
COMMON NAME: mugwort, little dragon.
OCCURRENCE: cultivated in kitchen gardens across Europe and Great Britain. Tarragon originally arose from both Siberia and southern Europe to form the French and Russian tarragon we know today.
PARTS USED: the leaves, which contain an essential volatile oil which is lost on drying.
MEDICINAL USES: today there are few medicinal uses for tarragon but it has been used previously to stimulate the appetite and to cure toothache. Tarragon is mostly used in cooking—particularly on the European continent. It is used for dressings, salads, vinegar and pickles.
ADMINISTERED AS: fresh root, fresh herb.

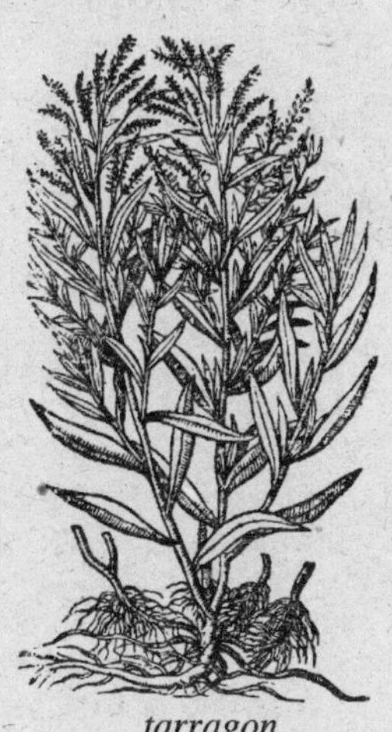
tarragon

Tea *Camellia thea.*
Common name: *Camellia theifera, Thea sinensis, Thea veridis, Thea bohea, Thea stricta jassamica.*
Occurrence: native to Assam in India, and the plant has spread to Sri Lanka, Java, China and Japan.
Parts used: the dried leaves.
Medicinal uses: stimulant, astringent. The infusion of the leaves has a stimulating effect on the nervous system, producing a feeling of comfort. It may also act as a nerve sedative where it can relieve headaches. When drunk in excessive quantities, tea can produce unpleasant nervous symptoms, dyspepsia and unnatural wakefulness.
Administered as: infusion.

Thistle, Holy *Carbenia benedicta.*
Common name: blessed thistle, *Cnicus benedictus, Carduus benedictus.*
Occurrence: a native of southern Europe and has been cultivated in Britain for hundreds of years.
Parts used: the whole herb which contains a volatile oil, a bitter crystalline compound called cnicin which is said to be similar to salicin in its properties.
Medicinal uses: tonic, stimulant, diaphoretic, emetic and emmenagogue. Very useful as an infusion to weak and debilitating stomach conditions, creating appetite and preventing sickness. It is said to be good in all fevers, as a purifier of the blood and circulation and its main modern day use is for bringing on a proper supply of milk in nursing mothers. In large doses, however, holy thistle is a strong emetic, producing vomiting. It may be used as a vermifuge.
Administered as: infusion and fluid extract.

Thistle, Scotch *Onopordon acanthium.*

COMMON NAME: woolly thistle, cotton thistle.

OCCURRENCE: a common plant in all of Great Britain, found in waste ground and roadsides.

PARTS USED: the leaves and root.

MEDICINAL USES: ancient herbalists believed that the Scotch thistle was a specific against cancer and even today the expressed juice of the plant has been used to good effect on cancers and ulcers. A decoction of thistles was thought to restore a healthy, growing head of hair when applied to a bald head, while a root decoction has astringent effects and reduces production from mucous membranes. Thistles were also supposed to be effective against rickets in children, a crick in the neck and nervous complaints.

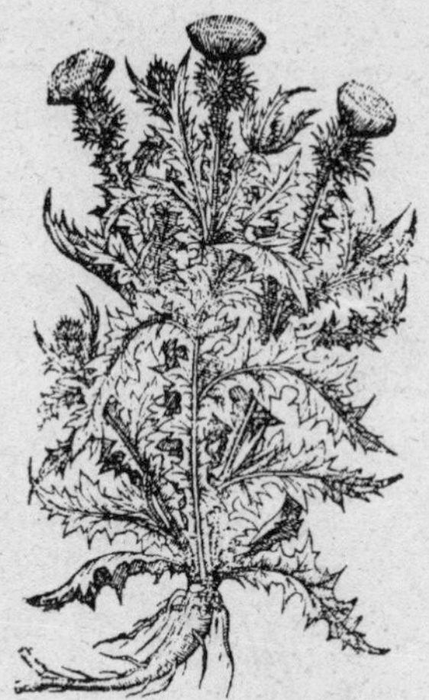

Scotch thistle

ADMINISTERED AS: expressed juice, decoction.

Thyme *Thymus vulgaris.*

COMMON NAME: garden or common thyme, tomillo.

OCCURRENCE: cultivated in temperate countries in northern Europe.

PARTS USED: the herb. Thyme gives rise to oil of thyme after distillation of the fresh leaves. This oil contains the phenols, thymol and carvacrol, as well as cymene, pinene and borneol.

MEDICINAL USES: antiseptic, antispasmodic, tonic, carminative. The fresh herb, in syrup, forms a safe cure for whooping cough, as is

an infusion of the dried herb. The infusion or tea is beneficial for catarrh, sore throat, wind spasms, colic and in allaying fevers and colds. Thyme is generally used in conjunction with other remedies in herbal medicine.
ADMINISTERED AS: fluid extract, essential oil and infusion.

Tobacco *Nicotiana tabacum, N. acuminata, N. rustica* and other varieties.
COMMON NAME: leaf tobacco, tabacca.
OCCURRENCE: native to America and cultivated in many sub-tropical countries including China, Greece, France and Turkey.
PARTS USED: the cured and dried leaves, which contain five alkaloids including nicotine. Upon smoking, nicotine decomposes into various chemicals—the very poisonous carbon monoxide, pyridine and hydrogen cyanide.
MEDICINAL USES: narcotic, sedative, diuretic, expectorant, emetic. Medicinally, tobacco has been used internally for hernias, constipation, tetanus, retention of urine, worms and hysterical convulsions. It is best utilized externally as a plaster or poultice to ease cutaneous diseases, haemorrhoids and facial neuralgia. A combination of tobacco leaves along with the leaves of STRAMONIUM or BELLADONNA make a very good treatment for spasmodic afflictions, painful tumours and obstinate ulcers. Tobacco is a local irritant and the nicotine within it is very

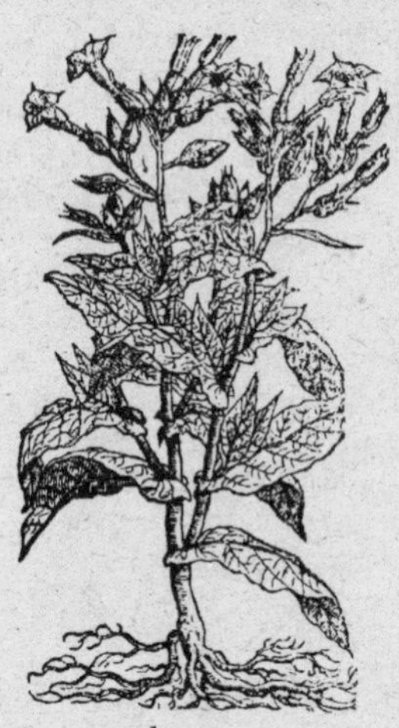

tobacco

poisonous, causing heart palpitations and irregularity and disturbing the digestive and circulatory organs. The use of tobacco as a medicine is unusual in today's western herbal medicine, although it is still used in some native societies. The poisonous nature of the alkaloids within the plant have discouraged its use as use of tobacco, even within small doses, can cause depression, convulsions and even death.
ADMINISTERED AS: poultice, ointment, suppositories, smoking herb.

Tree of heaven *Ailanthus glandulosa.*
COMMON NAME: ailanto, vernis de Japan, Chinese sumach.
OCCURRENCE: indigenous to China and India, and is now cultivated through Europe and the United State.
PARTS USED: the root and the inner bark of the tree. The bark contains chlorophyll, pectin, lignin, volatile oil, resin, quassin, tannin and various mineral salts.
MEDICINAL USES: astringent, antispasmodic, cardiac depressant. Despite this herb's unpleasant and nauseating action on patients, it has been successful against diarrhoea, dysentery, leucorrhoea, prolapse of the rectum and for tapeworms. A tincture prepared from the root bark of the tree has been good for epilepsy, asthma and cardiac palpitations.
ADMINISTERED AS: infusion, tincture.

Turpentine oil distilled from *Pinus palustris*, *Pinus maritima* and other species.
MEDICINAL USES: rubefacient, irritant, diuretic. When taken internally, turpentine forms a valuable remedy in bladder, kidney, and rheumatic problems and diseases of the mucous membranes. The oil is also used for respiratory complaints and externally as a liniment, an embrocation and an inhalant for rheumatism and chest

problems. Turpentine may be combined with other aromatic oils as a remedy.
ADMINISTERED AS: essential oil.

Valerian *Valeriana officinalis.*
COMMON NAME: all-heal, great wild valerian, amantilla, setwall, setewale, capon's tail.
OCCURRENCE: found throughout Europe and northern Asia. It is common in England in marshy thickets, riverbanks and ditches.
PARTS USED: the root, which contains a volatile oil, two alkaloids called chatarine and valerianine as well as several unidentified compounds.
MEDICINAL USES: powerful nervine, stimulant, carminative anodyne and antispasmodic herb. It may be given in all cases of nervous debility and irritation as it is not narcotic. The expressed juice of the fresh root has been used as a narcotic in insomnia and as an anticonvulsant in epilepsy. The oil of valerian is of use against cholera and in strengthening the eyesight. A herbal compound containing valerian was given to civilians during the Second World War, to reduce the effects of stress caused by repeated air raids and to minimize damage to health.
ADMINISTERED AS: fluid and solid extract, tincture, oil, expressed juice.

Verbena, Lemon *Lippia citriodora.*
COMMON NAME: herb Louisa, lemon-scented verbena, *Verveine citronelle* or *odorante*, *Verbena triphylla*, *Lippia triphylla*, *Aloysia citriodora.*
OCCURRENCE: originally from Peru and Chile, it was introduced into England in 1784 and is now a common garden plant.
PARTS USED: the leaves and flowering tops.
MEDICINAL USES: febrifuge, sedative. This herb has similar uses to

BALM, PEPPERMINT, ORANGE flowers and SPEARMINT in relieving flatulence, indigestion and dyspepsia through its antispasmodic and stomachic actions. It is commonly made into a refreshing tisane. The leaves of lemon verbena were once used in finger bowls at banquets and the essential oil distilled from the herb was used to impart a strong lemon scent to cosmetics and soaps.
ADMINISTERED AS: tea.

Vervain *Verbena officinalis.*
COMMON NAME: herb of grace, herbe sacrée, herba veneris, *Verbena hastrata.*
OCCURRENCE: grows across Europe, China, Japan and Barbary. Also found in England by roadsides and in sunny pastures.
PARTS USED: the herb. Vervain contains a peculiar tannin, which has not yet been fully investigated.
MEDICINAL USES: nervine, tonic, emetic, sudorific, astringent, diaphoretic, antispasmodic. This herb is recommended in many complaints including intermittent fevers, ulcers, pleurisy, ophthalmic disorders and is said to be a good galactogogue. May also be administered as a poultice to ease headache, ear neuralgia, rheumatism and taken as a decoction to ease bowel pain during purging. Vervain is often applied externally for piles.
ADMINISTERED AS: fluid extract, decoction.

Vine *Vitis vinifera.*
COMMON NAME: grape vine.
OCCURRENCE: a very ancient plant, frequently mentioned in the Bible after the Great Flood. It now grows in Asia, central and southern Europe, Africa, Australia, Greece, California and South America.
PARTS USED: the fruit, leaves and juice. The wine sold commercially is made from fermented fruit juice. This juice, which is called

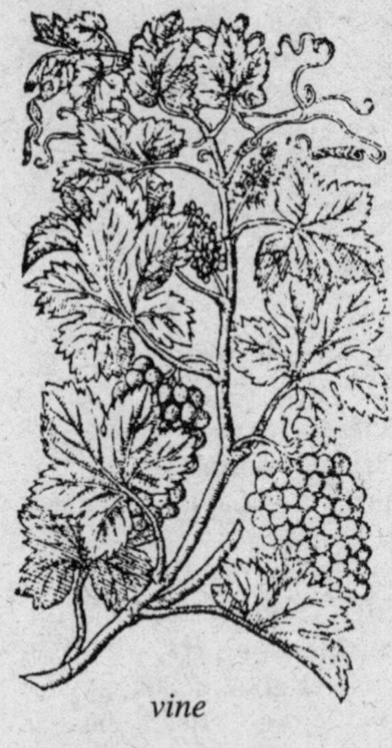
vine

'must', contains malic acid, gum, sugar, inorganic salts and potassium bicarbonate. The leaves contain tartaric acid, tannin, malic acid, gum, quercetine, quercitrin, potassium bitartrate, cane sugar and glucose.

MEDICINAL USES: the leaves and seeds have an astringent action, with the leaves previously used to stop haemorrhages and bleeding. Ripe grapes, when eaten in some quantity, increase the flow of urine and can be of great benefit in exhaustion, anaemia, smallpox, sleeplessness and neuralgia. They are also eaten for poor biliary function and torpid liver. Grape sugar is chemically different to other sugars, as the saliva has no enzymatic effect on it. Thus it acts faster to warm up the body and build tissues, to increase strength and repair the body after illness. Raisins have demulcent, nutritive and slightly laxative effects on the body.

ADMINISTERED AS: fermented fruit juice, fresh or dried leaves, fresh or dried fruits.

Violet *Viola adorata.*

COMMON NAME: blue violet, sweet violet, sweet-scented violet.

OCCURRENCE: native to Great Britain and found widely over Europe, northern Asia and North America.

PARTS USED: the dried flowers and leaves and whole plant when fresh.

MEDICINAL USES: antiseptic, expectorant, laxative. The herb is mainly taken as syrup of violets which has been used to cure the ague, epilepsy, eye inflammation, pleurisy, jaundice and sleeplessness which are some of the many other complaints that benefit from treatment with this herb. The flowers possess expectorant properties and have long been used to treat coughs. The flowers may also be crystallized as a sweetmeat or added to salads. The rhizome is strongly emetic and purgative and has violent effects when administered. The seeds also have purgative and diuretic effects and are beneficial in treating urinary complaints and gravel. In the early part of this century, violet preparations were used to great effect against cancer. Fresh violet leaves are made into an infusion which was drunk regularly, and a poultice of the leaves was applied to the affected area. The herb has been used successfully to both allay pain and perhaps cure the cancer. It is said to be particularly good against throat cancer.
ADMINISTERED AS: infusion, poultice, injection, ointment, syrup and powdered root.

Walnut *Juglans nigra.*
COMMON NAME: carya, Jupiter's nuts, *Juglans regia.*
OCCURRENCE: cultivated throughout Europe and was probably native to Persia.
PARTS USED: the bark and leaves. The active principle of the walnut tree is nucin or juglon, while the kernels also contain oil, mucilage, albumin, cellulose, mineral matter and water.
MEDICINAL USES: alterative, laxative, detergent, astringent. The bark and leaves are used in skin problems, e.g. scrofulous diseases, herpes, eczema and for healing indolent ulcers. A strong infusion of the powdered bark has purgative effects, while the walnut has various properties dependent upon its stage of ripeness. Green walnuts are anthelminthic and vermifuge in action and are pickled in

vinegar, which is then used as a gargle for sore and ulcerated throats. The wood is used for furniture, gun-stocks and for cabinets. Walnut oil expressed from the kernels is used in wood polishing, painting and is used as butter or frying oil.
Administered as: fluid extract, infusion, expressed oil, whole fruit.

Water betony *Scrophularia aquatica.*
Common name: water figwort, brownwort, bishop's leaves, crowdy kit, fiddlewood, fiddler, *Betonica aquatica.*
Occurrence: found growing wild in damp places, on the banks of rivers and ponds throughout Great Britain and Europe.
Parts used: the leaves, fresh and dried.
Medicinal uses: detergent, vulnerary. The leaves are used as a poultice, or as an ointment for wounds, sores, haemorrhoids, ulcers and scrofulous glands in the neck. It was also used to expel nightmares, cure toothache and as a cosmetic for blemished or sunburnt skin.
Administered as: decoction, poultice, ointment.

Watercress *Nasturtium officinale*
Occurrence: a perennial creeping plant often growing near springs and running water across Great Britain and Europe.
Parts used: the stem and leaves, which contain nicotinamide, volatile oil, a glucoside, gluconasturtin and vitamins A, C and E.
Medicinal uses: stimulant, expectorant, nutritive, antiscorbutic, diuretic. Watercress was proposed as a specific in tuberculosis and has a very long history of medical use. It is used to treat bronchitis and coughs as well as boosting digestion, lowering blood sugar and helping the body to remove toxic wastes from the blood and tissues. The herb is of value nutritionally as it contains many vitamins and mineral salts which help during conva-

lescence and general debility. It can be bruised and made into a poultice for arthritis and gout, and is chewed raw to strengthen gums.
ADMINISTERED AS: expressed juice, poultice, dietary item.

Water dock *Rumex aquaticus.*
COMMON NAME: red dock, bloodwort.
OCCURRENCE: found frequently in fields, meadows, pools and ditches throughout Europe and Great Britain and is particularly common in the northern latitudes.
PARTS USED: the root.
MEDICINAL USES: alterative, deobstruent, detergent. It has a powerful tonic action and is used externally to clean ulcers in afflictions of the mouth. It is applied to eruptive and scorbutic diseases, skin ulcers and sores. As a powder, Water dock has a cleansing and detergent effect upon the teeth.
ADMINISTERED AS: fluid extract and infusion.

Willow, White *Salix alba.*
COMMON NAME: European willow.
OCCURRENCE: a large tree growing in moist places and running streams around Great Britain and Europe.
PARTS USED: the bark and leaves. The bark contains tannin and salicin.
MEDICINAL USES: tonic, antiperiodic, astringent. The bark has been used in febrile diseases of rheumatic or gouty origin, diarrhoea and dysentery. It has been used in dyspepsia connected with digestive organ disorders. The bark has also been of benefit in convalescence after acute diseases and against parasitic worms.
ADMINISTERED AS: decoction, powdered root.

Wintergreen *Gaultheria procumbens*.
COMMON NAME: mountain tea, teaberry, boxberry, thé du Canada, aromatic wintergreen, partridge berry, deerberry, checkerberry.
OCCURRENCE: native to the northern United States and Canada from Georgia northwards.
PARTS USED: the leaves, which produce a volatile oil upon distillation. The oil is made up of methyl salicylate, gaultherilene, an aldehyde, a secondary alcohol and an ester. The aromatic odour of the plant is due to the alcohol and the ester.
MEDICINAL USES: aromatic, tonic, stimulant, diuretic, emmenagogue, astringent, galactogogue. The oil is of great benefit in acute rheumatism, but must be given in the form of capsules so stomach inflammation does not occur. The true distilled oil when applied to the skin can give rise to an eruption and so the synthetic oil of wintergreen is recommended for external use as it still contains methyl salicylate, but with no deleterious effects. The synthetic oil is exceedingly valuable for all chronic joint and muscular troubles, lumbago, sciatica and rheumatism. The oil is also used as a flavouring for toothpowders and mouth washes, particularly when combined with menthol and EUCALYPTUS. The berries are a winter food for many animals and also produce a bitter tonic, after being steeped in brandy. The leaves are either used to flavour tea or as a substitute for tea itself.
ADMINISTERED AS: capsules, synthetic oil, infusion, tincture.

Witch hazel *Hamamelis virginiana*.
COMMON NAME: spotted alder, winterbloom, snapping hazelnut.
OCCURRENCE: native to the United States of America and Canada.
PARTS USED: the dried bark, both fresh and dried leaves. The leaves contain tannic and gallic acids, volatile oil and an unknown bitter

principle. The bark contains tannin, gallic acid, a physterol, resin, fat and other bitter and odorous bodies.

MEDICINAL USES: astringent, tonic, sedative. Valuable in stopping internal and external haemorrhages and in treating piles. Mainly used for bruises, swelling, inflammation and tumours as a poultice. It may also be utilized for diarrhoea, dysentery and mucous discharges. A decoction is used against tuberculosis, gonorrhoea, menorrhagia and the debilitated state resulting from abortion. Tea made from the bark or leaves aids bleeding of the stomach, bowel complaints and may be given as an injection for bleeding piles. Witch hazel is used to treat varicose veins as a moist poultice, as an extract to ease burns, scalds and insect and mosquito bites, and to help inflammation of the eyelids.

ADMINISTERED AS: liquid extract, injection, tincture, lotion, ointment, suppositories, poultice, infusion and decoction.

Woodruff *Asperula odorata.*

COMMON NAME: wuderove, wood-rova, sweet woodruff, woodroof, waldmeister tea.

OCCURRENCE: grows in woods or shaded hedges in England.

PARTS USED: the herb, which contains coumarin, a fragrant crystalline chemical, citric, malic and rubichloric acids and tannic acid.

MEDICINAL USES: diuretic, tonic. The fresh leaves, when applied to wounds, were said to have a strong healing effect. A strong decoction of the fresh herb was used as a cordial and stomachic and is said to be useful in removing biliary obstructions of the liver.

ADMINISTERED AS: a poultice and decoction.

Wormseed, American *Chenopodium anthelminticum.*

COMMON NAME: Mexican tea, Jesuit's tea, herba Sancti Mariae, *Chenopodium ambrosioides.*

OCCURRENCE: indigenous to Mexico and South America, and naturalized in almost all areas of the eastern United States.
PARTS USED: the fruits and seeds. An oil is distilled from the crushed fruits called chenopodium oil. It is made up of ascaridole, an unstable substance, choline, betzine, sylvestrene and several other compounds.
MEDICINAL USES: anthelmintic, vermifuge. The herb is used to expel roundworms and hookworms, particularly in children. The drug should be given in one full dose, then fasting until an active purgative drug e.g. CASTOR OIL is given two hours later. The treatment should be repeated ten days later. The drug may be given as volatile oil, expressed juice of the fresh plant, the fluid extract, or the bruised fruit. Chenopodium oil has been of benefit in chorea, malaria, hysteria and similar nervous diseases and has been used as a pectoral drug in asthma and catarrh. Unfortunately the chenopodium oil on the market varies as to the quantity of ascaridole within it and care must be taken to prevent overdoses occurring. Toxic symptoms caused by this drug include temporary dizziness and vomiting.
ADMINISTERED AS: distilled oil, expressed juice, bruised fruit, fluid extract.

Wormwood *Artemisia absinthium.*
COMMON NAME: green ginger, old women, ajenjo.
OCCURRENCE: a plant found wild in many parts of the world including Siberia, Europe and the United States of America.
PARTS USED: the whole herb. The herb contains a volatile oil made up of thujone, pinene, cadinene and chamazulene, a bitter principle called absinthum, carotene, tannins and vitamin C.
MEDICINAL USES: bitter tonic, anthelmintic, febrifuge, stomachic. The liqueur, absinthe, was made using this plant as flavouring and it was banned in France in 1915 as excess intake caused

irreversible damage to the nervous system. In modern herbal medicine, it is used as a bitter tonic to stimulate the appetite, the liver and gall bladder, production of digestive juices and peristalsis. Wormwood also expels parasitic worms, particularly roundworms and threadworms. The plant contains chemicals which have anti-inflammatory effects and help reduce fevers. Since ancient times this herb has been used by women to encourage menstruation, and it is applied as an external compress during labour to speed up the birth process. After labour, wormwood was taken both internally and externally to expel the afterbirth. This herb should not be used during pregnancy and should only be administered for short time periods.
ADMINISTERED AS: infusion, essential oil, fluid extract.

Woundwort *Stachys palustris*.
COMMON NAME: all-heal, panay, opopanewort, clown's woundwort, rusticum vulna herba, downy woundwort, stinking marsh stachys.
OCCURRENCE: common to marshy meadows, riversides and ditches in most parts of Great Britain.
PARTS USED: the herb.
MEDICINAL USES: antiseptic, antispasmodic. The herb relieves cramp, gout, painful joints and vertigo, while bruised leaves will stop bleeding and encourage healing when applied to a wound. Woundwort had an excellent reputation as a vulnerary among all of the early herbalists. A syrup made of the fresh juice will stop haemorrhages and dysentery when taken internally. The tuberous roots are edible as are the young shoot which resemble ASPARAGUS.
ADMINISTERED AS: poultice or syrup.

Yam, wild *dioscorea villosa.*
COMMON NAME: dioscorea, colic root, rheumatism root, wilde yamwurzel.
OCCURRENCE: native to the southern United States and Canada.
PARTS USED: the roots and rhizome, which contain steroidal saponins, phytosterols, tannins, starch and various alkaloids including dioscorine.
MEDICINAL USES: antispasmodic, diuretic. This plant has a history of traditional use in relieving menstrual cramps and in stopping threatened miscarriage. It brings quick relief for bilious colic and flatulence, particularly in pregnant women. It is prescribed for the inflammatory stage of rheumatoid arthritis and in painful disorders of the urinary tract. Wild Yam is also beneficial for poor circulation, spasmodic hiccoughs, neuralgic complaints and spasmodic asthma. Prior to 1970, the wild yam was the only source of diosgenin, one of the starting materials used in commercial manufacturing of steroid hormones for the contraceptive pill.
ADMINISTERED AS: fluid extract, powdered bark, infusion.

Yerba santa *Eriodictyon glutinosum.*
COMMON NAME: mountain balm, gum bush, bear's weed, holy or sacred herb, consumptive's weed, *Eriodictyon californicum.*
OCCURRENCE: native to California and northern Mexico.
PARTS USED: the dried leaves which contain five phenolic chemicals, free acids including free formic acids, volatile oil, phytosterol, glucose, a resin and some glycerides of fatty acids.
MEDICINAL USES: bitter tonic, stimulant, expectorant, aromatic. This herb is recommended in laryngeal and bronchial problems, catarrh, hay fever, asthma and chronic lung afflictions. It is also used for catarrh of the bladder and haemorrhoids. Yerba santa is used as a bitter tonic upon the digestion and is highly effective in masking the unpleasant taste of quinine,

when given as an aromatic syrup. The dried leaves are smoked to ease asthma.
ADMINISTERED AS: powdered leaves, fluid extract, syrup.

Yew *Taxus baccata.*
OCCURRENCE: found in Europe, North Africa and Western Asia. The tree has been closely associated with the history and legends of Europe.
PARTS USED: the leaves, seeds and fruit. The seeds and fruit are the most poisonous parts of the plant and contain an alkaloid toxine and another principle milrossin.
MEDICINAL USES: it has few medicinal uses due to its poisonous nature but the leaves were once used effectively in treating epilepsy. The wood was used for making longbows.
ADMINISTERED AS: powdered leaves.

Herb Action

alterative a term given to a substance that speeds up the renewal of the tissues so that they can carry out their functions more effectively.

anodyne a drug that eases and soothes pain.

anthelmintic a substance that causes the death or expulsion of parasitic worms.

antiperiodic a drug that prevents the return of recurring diseases, e.g. malaria.

antiscorbutic a substance that prevents scurvy and contains necessary vitamins, e.g. vitamin C.

antiseptic a substance that prevents the growth of disease-causing micro-organisms, e.g. bacteria, without causing damage to living tissue. It is applied to wounds to cleanse them and prevent infection.

antispasmodic a drug that diminishes muscle spasms.

aperient a medicine that produces a natural movement of the bowel.

aphrodisiac a compound that excites the sexual organs.

aromatic a substance that has an aroma.

astringent a substance that causes cells to contract by losing proteins from their surface. This causes localized contraction of blood vessels and tissues.

balsamic a substance that contains resins and benzoic acid and is used to alleviate colds and abrasions.

bitter a drug that is bitter-tasting and is used to stimulate the appetite.

cardiac compounds that have some effect on the heart.

carminative a preparation to relieve flatulence and any resultant griping.

cathartic a compound that produces an evacuation of the bowels.

cholagogue the name given to a substance that produces a flow of bile from the gall bladder.

cooling a substance that reduces the temperature and cools the skin.

demulcent a substance that soothes and protects the alimentary canal.

deobstruent a compound that is said to clear obstructions and open the natural passages of the body.

detergent a substance that has a cleansing action, either internally or on the skin.

diaphoretic a term given to drugs that promote perspiration.

diuretics a substance that stimulates the kidneys and increases urine and solute production.

emetic a drug that induces vomiting.

emmenagogue a compound that is able to excite the menstrual discharge.

emollient a substance that softens or soothes the skin.

expectorant a group of drugs that are taken to help in the removal of secretions from the lungs, bronchi and trachea.

febrifuge a substance that reduces fever.

galactogogue an agent that stimulates the production of breast milk or increases milk flow.

haemostatic a drug used to control bleeding.

hepatic a substance that acts upon the liver.

hydrogogue a substance that has the property of removing accumulations of water or serum.

hypnotic a drug or substance that induces sleep.

insecticide a substance that kills insects.

irritant a general term encompassing any agent that causes irritation of a tissue.

laxative a substance that is taken to evacuate the bowel or soften stools.

mydriatic a compound that causes dilation of the pupil.

nervine a name given to drugs that are used to restore the nerves to their natural state.

narcotic a drug that leads to stupor and complete loss of awareness.

nephritic a drug that has an action on the kidneys.

nutritive a compound that is nourishing to the body.

parasiticide a substance that destroys parasites internally and externally.

pectoral a term applied to drugs that are remedies in treating chest and lung complaints.

purgative the name given to drugs or other measures that produce evacuation of the bowels. They normally have a more severe effect than aperients or laxatives.

refrigerant a substance that relieves thirst and produces a feeling of coolness.

resolvent a substance that is applied to swellings to reduce them in size.

rubefacient a compound that causes the skin to redden and peel off. It causes blisters and inflammation.

sedative a drug that lessens tension, anxiety and soothes over-excitement of the nervous system.

sternutatory the name given to a substance that irritates the mucous membrane and produces sneezing.

stimulant a drug or other agent that increases the activity of an organ or system within the body.

stomachic name given to drugs that treat stomach disorders.

styptic applications that check bleeding by blood vessel contraction or by causing rapid blood clotting.

sudorific a drug or agent that produces copious perspiration.
taeniacide drugs that are used to expel tapeworms from the body.
tonic substances that are traditionally thought to give strength and vigour to the body and that are said to produce a feeling of well-being.
vermifuge a substance that kills, or expels, worms from the intestines.
vesicant similar to a rubefacient, agent that causes blistering when applied to the skin.
vulnerary a drug that is said to be good at healing wounds.

Classification of Herbs by Action

alterative anemone pulsatilla, bethroot, betony (wood), bitter root, bittersweet, blue flag, brooklime, burdock, burr marigold, caroba, celandine, clivers, clover (red), cohosh (black), dock (yellow), dropwort (water), echinacea, elder, fireweed, fringe tree, frostwort, golden seal, Jacob's ladder, meadowsweet, mezeron, pipsissewa, plantain (common), poke root, polypody root, rosinweed, sarsaparilla (Jamaica), sassafras, soap tree, soapwort, speedwell, spindle tree, tag alder, walnut.

anodyne aconite, camphor, chamomile, coca, figwort, gladwyn, henbane, hemlock, hops, hound's tongue, lettuce (wild), mandrake, poppy (red), poppy (white), sassy bark, stramonium, valerian.

anthelmintic aloes, balmony, camphor, cedar (yellow), cohosh (blue), gentian (yellow), groundsel, hellebore (black), knotgrass, lupin (white), male fern, savine, tansy, walnut, wormseed (American), wormwood.

antiperiodic lilac, willow (white).

antiscorbutic groundsel, lemon, lime fruit, radish, rowan tree, scurvy grass, shepherd's purse, sorrel, spinach, watercress.

antiseptic avens, barberry, beech, bergamot, bethroot, black root, camphor, cinnamon, costmary, echinacea, elecampane, eucalyptus, garlic, gentian (yellow), horseradish, myrrh, oak, olive, sandalwood, stockholm tar, thyme, violet, woundwort.

antispasmodic anemone pulsatilla, arrach, baneberry, belladonna, bergamot, camphor, chamomile, clover (red), cohosh (blue), cowslip, cramp bark, cumin, daisy (ox-eye), ephedra, eucalyptus, gelsemium, gladwyn, hemlock, henbane, masterwort, mayweed, mistletoe, motherwort, musk seed, oats, passionflower, peony, peppermint, pleurisy root, poppy (white), primrose, red root, rosinweed, rue, scullcap (Virginian), skunk-cabbage, spearmint, stramonium, sumbul, thyme, tree of heaven, valerian, vervain, woundwort, yam (wild).

aperient butcher's broom, clivers, club moss, costmary, couchgrass, dandelion, elder, feverfew, fringe tree, fumitory, germander (wall), horseradish, jewelweed, olive, parsley, rhubarb, rose (pale), scurvy grass.

aphrodisiac celery, coca, damiana, guarana, musk seed.

aromatic allspice, angelica, angostura, asarabacca, avens, basil, bergamot, betony (wood), birthwort, bugle, calamint, calamus, camphor, caraway, cardamom, cedar (yellow), cicely (sweet), cinnamon, cloves, coriander, dill, eryngo, eucalyptus, fennel, gale (sweet), golden rod, hops, lavender, lovage, magnolia, meadowsweet, melilot, musk seed, orange (bitter), orange (sweet), pepper, pine oils, sage (common), St. John's wort, sandalwood, sassafras, savory (summer), saxifrage (burnet), spearmint, wintergreen, yerba santa.

astringent agrimony, alder, apple, avens, bayberry, bearberry, bethroot, betony (wood), birch, bistort, blackberry, bugle, burnet (greater), cassia, cedar (yellow), chestnut (horse), chestnut (sweet), cinnamon, cohosh (black), columbine, comfrey, costmary, cudweed, dog-rose, elder, elecampane, elm, evening primrose, eyebright, fireweed, frostwort, gale (sweet), golden rod, hawthorn, horsetail, hound's tongue, houseleek, ivy (ground), Jacob's ladder, knotgrass, lady's mantle, larch, lily (Madonna), loosestrife, lungwort, maple (red), matico, meadowsweet, mullein, myrrh, nettle, oak, olive, pipsissewa, plantain (common), poppy (white), primrose, quince, ragwort, raspberry, red root, rhubarb, rose (pale), rose (red), rosemary, rowan tree, rupturewort, sage (common), sassy bark, scullcap (Virginian), self-heal, St. John's wort, silverweed, solomon's seal, speedwell (common), strawberry, tag alder, tea, thistle (scotch), tree of heaven, vervain, vine, walnut, willow (white), wintergreen, witch hazel.

balsamic larch.

bitter angostura, bugle, birch, calumba, feverfew, gentian (yellow), nux vomica, simaruba, snapdragon, wormwood, yerba santa.

cardiac asparagus, bitter root, butterbur, foxglove, hawthorn, kola nuts, lily of the valley, mescal buttons, strophanthus, tree of heaven.

carminative allspice, angelica, anise, balm, basil, bergamot, calamus, caraway, cardamom, cassia, catmint, cayenne, celery, cicely (sweet), cinnamon, cloves, coriander, cumin, dill, fennel, feverfew, ginger, golden rod, horsemint (American), juniper, lavender, lovage, mace, marjoram, masterwort, melilot, nutmeg, orange (bitter), orange (sweet), parsley, pennyroyal, pepper, peppermint, pleurisy root, saffron, sage (common), savory (summer), saxifrage (burnet), spearmint, thyme, valerian.

cathartic black root, bloodroot, blue flag, bogbean, broom, bryony (white), castor oil plant, croton, fireweed, gladwyn, hedge-hyssop, hydrangea, ivy, jewelweed, mountain flax, pleurisy root, poke root, sabadilla, saffron (meadow), senna, stavesacre.

cholagogue spindle tree.

cooling basil, cucumber, lemon, mandrake, plantain (common), ragwort, sorrel, witch hazel.

demulcent almonds, barley, borage, chickweed, coltsfoot, comfrey, couchgrass, elm, fig, flax, hound's tongue, Iceland moss, Irish moss, lily (Madonna), liquorice, marshmallow, mullein, olive, parsley piert, peach, pellitory-of-the-wall, pine (white), pumpkin, quince, rice, salep, slippery elm, Solomon's seal, sundew.

deobstruent agrimony, bladderwrack, bogbean, butcher's broom, carrot, liverwort (English), plantain (common), water dock.

depurative figwort.

detergent balmony, blackcurrant, golden seal, ragwort, soap tree, soapwort, walnut, water betony, water dock.

diaphoretic aconite, anemone pulsatilla, angelica, balm, blackcurrant, black root, boneset, box, buchu, burdock, burr marigold, butcher's broom, camphor, caroba, carrot, catmint, chicory, clematis, clivers, cohosh (blue), cuckoopint, dwarf elder, elder, elecampane, eryngo, fumitory, garlic, gelsemium, germander (wall), groundsel, heartease, hedge-hyssop, horehound, horsemint (American), horseradish, ipecacuanha, ivy, jaborandi, Jacob's ladder, knapweed (greater), laurel, lettuce (wild), lily of the valley, lobelia, lovage, marigold, marjoram, motherwort, mugwort, pennyroyal, pimpernel (scarlet), pine (white), pleurisy root, poppy (white), ragwort, rosemary, rosinweed, saffron, samphire, sarsaparilla (Jamaica), sassafras, saxifrage (burnet), senega, sheep's sorrel, skunk-cabbage, slippery elm, smartweed, speedwell (common), stockholm tar, thistle (holy), turpentine, vervain, woodruff.

diuretic apple, arnica, asparagus, belladonna, bittersweet, blackcurrant, blue flag, bluebell, broom, buchu, burdock, burr marigold, butterbur, cacao, caroba, cedar (yellow), celandine, celery, clematis, club moss, coffee, cohosh (black), cohosh (blue), coolwort, couchgrass, cucumber, daisy (ox-eye), damiana, dandelion, dropwort (water), dwarf elder, elder, elm, eryngo, figwort, foxglove, fringe tree, fumitory, garlic, germander (wall), golden rod, groundsel, goutwort, hair cup moss, hawthorn, heartease, henbane, hops, horsemint (American), horseradish, horsetail, houseleek, hydrangea, ivy (ground), jewelweed, juniper, kava-kava, knotgrass, kola nuts, larch, lettuce (wild), lupin (white), mastic, matico, meadowsweet, mezeron, mugwort, mustard (black), nettle, parsley, parsley piert, peach, pellitory-of-the-wall, pimpernel (scarlet), pipsissewa, plantain (common), poplar, pumpkin, radish, rest-harrow, rosinweed, rupturewort, sandalwood, sarsaparilla (jamaica), sassafras, savine, saw palmetto, saxifrage (burnet), scurvy grass, senega, sheep's sorrel, shepherd's purse, smartweed, soap tree, sorrel, St. John's wort, stockholm tar, strawberry, sunflower, tobacco, vine, watercress, wintergreen, yam (wild).

emetic asarabacca, black root, bloodroot, daffodil, elder, fireweed, groundsel, hedge-hyssop, ipecacuanha, jewelweed, laurel, lobelia, mandrake, mayweed, mescal buttons, mustard (black), poke root, primrose, rosinweed, sabadilla, saffron (meadow), spearwort (lesser), stavesacre, tag alder, thistle (holy), tobacco, vervain.

emmenagogue aloes, arrach, bloodroot, cassia, catmint, cedar (yellow), cohosh (black), cohosh (blue), cornflower, cotton root, ergot, feverfew, gale (sweet), gentian (yellow), hellebore (black), horsemint (American), lupin (white), marjoram, marjoram (sweet), mayweed, motherwort, mugwort, myrrh, pennyroyal, rue, saffron, savine, senega, smartweed, tansy, thistle (holy), wintergreen.

emollient almonds, borage, cacao, cucumber, fenugreek, fig, flax, Irish moss, liquorice, marshmallow, melilot, mullein, olive, ragwort, slippery elm.

expectorant balsam of Peru, beech, bethroot, bloodroot, boneset, calamint, cedar (yellow), cicely (sweet), cohosh (black), coltsfoot, comfrey, cuckoopint, cup moss, dropwort (water), dwarf elder, elder, elecampane, eryngo, garlic, ginger, honeysuckle, horehound, ipecacuanha, jaborandi, Jacob's ladder, larch, lobelia, loosestrife, maidenhair, myrrh, peach, pimpernel (scarlet), pine (white), pleurisy root, polypody root, poppy (red), poppy (white), red root, rosinweed, St. John's wort, senega, skunk-cabbage, slippery elm, soap tree, speedwell (common), stockholm tar, sundew, sunflower, tobacco, violet, watercress, yerba santa.

febrifuge aconite, avens, balm, blackcurrant, bogbean, boneset, calumba, chestnut (horse), gelsemium, gentian (yellow), guarana, holly, lilac, pepper, poplar, verbena (lemon), wormwood.

galactogogue castor oil plant, vervain, wintergreen.

haemostatic puffballa, shepherd's purse.

hepatic dodder, spindle tree.

hydragogue bitter root, bryony (white).

hypnotic corkwood tree, henbane, mandrake, poppy (white).

insecticide laburnum, larkspur, musk weed, pyrethrum (dalmatian).

irritant bryony (white), cedar (yellow), croton, ivy (poison), mustard (black), pellitory, rue, turpentine.

laxative almonds, asparagus, boneset, castor oil plant, chicory, dock (yellow), dodder, elder, fig, golden seal, honeysuckle, mountain flax, mulberry, olive, pellitory-of-the-wall, rose (pale), sassy bark, senna, spinidle tree, strawberry, violet, walnut.

mydriatic belladonna, corkwood tree, henbane.

narcotic belladonna, bittersweet, box, cherry laurel, chestnut (horse), guarana, hellebore (black), henbane, ivy (poison), laurel, lettuce (wild), mescal buttons, mistletoe, mullein, nightshade (black), paris (herb), passionflower, poke root, poppy (red), sassy bark, skunk-cabbage, stramonium, tobacco.

nephritic hydrangea.

nervine anemone pulsatilla, arrach, celery, club moss, cramp bark, guarana, kola nuts, hops, lavender, lime tree, mistletoe, motherwort, mugwort, musk seed, oats, scullcap (Virginian), St. John's wort, sumbul, valerian, vervain.

nutritive almonds, barley, cacao, fig, Iceland moss, Irish moss, mulberry, oats, parsnip, rice, salep, saw palmetto, slippery elm, spinach, watercress.

parasiticide balsam of Peru, larkspur.

pectoral anise, bethroot, dog-rose, euphorbia, flax, horehound, Irish moss, liquorice, lungwort, maidenhair, polypody root, slippery elm, sundew.

purgative aloes, angostura, asarabacca, barberry, bindweed (greater), castor oil plant, celandine, croton, cucumber, damiana, dodder, dwarf elder, elder, groundsel, hellebore (black), kamala, liverwort (English), mandrake, mercury (dog's), mountain flax, rhubarb, senna.

refrigerant blackcurrant, borage, catmint, chickweed, dog-rose, houseleek, lemon, lime fruit, mulberry, parsley piert, pellitory-of-the-wall, plantain (common), rice, sheep's sorrel, sorrel.

resolvent bittersweet, saxifrage (burnet), St. John's wort.

rubefacient bryony (black), buttercup (bulbous), cayenne, croton, horsemint (American), horseradish, ivy (poison), pellitory, pine oils, rue, spearwort (lesser), turpentine.

sedative aconite, asparagus, belladonna, box, camphor, cherry laurel, clover (red), corkwood tree, cowslip, cramp bark, ergot, evening primrose, foxglove, gelsemium, goutwort, hemlock, henbane, lettuce (wild), motherwort, mullein, passionflower, peach, poppy (white), red root, saw palmetto, skunk-cabbage, tobacco, verbena (lemon), witch hazel.

sternulatory asarabacca, soap tree, soapwort.

stimulant allspice, angelica, angostura, arnica, asarabacca, balsam of Peru, bayberry, beech, birthwort, blue flag, boneset, buchu, butterbur, cacao, calamus, caraway, cardamom, carrot, catmint, cayenne, celery, chives, cinnamon, cloves, coca, coffee, coriander, cornflower, cuckoopint, cumin, damiana, dill, elder, elecampane, ephedra, ergot, eryngo, eucalyptus, fennel, feverfew, garlic, germander (wall), ginger, ginseng, golden rod, guarana, horsemint (American), horseradish, ipecacuanha, ivy, ivy (ground), ivy (poison), jabarandi, kava-kava, kola nuts, larch, lavender, lime tree, lobelia, lovage, mace, magnolia, marigold, marjoram, marjoram (sweet), masterwort, mastic, matico, mezeron, mugwort, mustard (black), myrrh, nettle, nutmeg, nux vomica, oats, pennyroyal, pepper, peppermint, poplar, raspberry, rosemary, rue, sage (common), sassafras, scurvy grass, senega, shepherd's purse, smartweed, snapdragon, soap tree, spearmint, spindle tree, stockholm tar, sumbul, tansy, tea, thistle (holy), valerian, watercress, wintergreen, yerba santa.

stomachic angelica, avens, cassia, chamomile, cicely (sweet), dill, fennel, gentian (yellow), ginseng, golden seal, juniper, laurel, musk seed, nutmeg, orange (bitter), orange (sweet), peppermint, rhubarb, saxifrage (burnet), wormwood.

styptic avens, bluebell, knotgrass, lady's mantle, matico, self-heal.

sudorific avens, nightshade (black), vervain.

taeniacide cucumber, kamala, male fern, pumpkin.

tonic agrimony, alder, angelica, angostura, asarabacca, avens, balmony, barberry, bayberry, bergamot, bethroot, bitter root, black root, blackberry, bogbean, boneset, burnet (greater), butterbur, calamus, calumba, cassia, catmint, cayenne, celery, chamomile, chestnut (horse), chestnut (sweet), chicory, clivers, coca, coltsfoot, coolwort, cornflower, daisy (ox-eye), damiana, dandelion, dock (yellow), elecampane, elm, eyebright, fireweed, foxglove, fringe tree, frostwort, fumitory, gentian (yellow), germander (wall), ginseng, golden seal, guarana, hawthorn, holly, hops, horehound, hydrangea, Iceland moss, ivy (ground), kava-kava, knapweed (greater), kola nuts, lemon, lilac, lily of the valley, lime tree, mace, magnolia, marjoram, marjoram (sweet), mayweed, mescal buttons, mistletoe, motherwort, mugwort, myrrh, nettle, nux vomica, oak, orange (bitter), orange (sweet), parsley, peony, pipsissewa, pleurisy root, polypody root, poplar, rose (red), rosemary, rosinweed, sage (common), sarsaparilla (Jamaica), saw palmetto, scullcap (Virginian), self-heal, silverweed, simaruba, soapwort, solomon's seal, speedwell (common), spindle tree, strophanthus, sumbul, tag alder, tansy, thistle (holy), thyme, vervain, willow (white), wintergreen, witch hazel, wormwood, woodruff, yerba santa.

vermifuge aloes, castor oil plant, cohosh (blue), lilac, male fern, pink root, primrose, sabadilla, stavesacre, walnut, wormseed (American).

vesicant mezereon.

vulnerary arnica, comfrey, knotgrass, mare's tail, water betony.

Chemical Glossary

acid a substance that can form hydrogen ions when dissolved in water. Aqueous solutions of acids typically have a sharp taste and turn litmus paper red. Most organic acids have the C(O)OH grouping but they may have other acid groups, e.g. the sulphonic group—$S(O_2)OH$. Acids can vary in strength according to the degree of ionization in solution.

alcohol an organic compound with one or more hydroxyl (-OH) groups attached directly to a carbon atom. This is a large assemblage of compounds that form part of waxes, esters, aldehydes, ketones and volatile oils. Alcohols may be in the solid or liquid form depending on the size of the carbon chain.

aldehydes organic compounds with a carbonyl group joined directly to another carbon atom. Aldehydes may be either solids or colourless liquids.

alkali the name given to a substance that gives a solution in water with a pH of greater than seven. They may also be called a base.

alkaloid probably the most important chemicals found in plants, as they usually have a medical action. They are organic substances, found in association with organic acids in most plant groups, particularly the flowering plants. Alkaloids are alkaline and combine with acids to form crystalline salts which are water-soluble in most cases. The alkaloids themselves are generally insoluble in water but dissolve well in alcohol or ether. Alkaloids include a number of important drugs, e.g. morphine, caffeine, atropine, quinine and nicotine and many of these chemicals are very poisonous with characteristic physiological effects.

anthraquinones glycoside compounds present in some plants and that are used to prepare dyes and purgative drugs.

bitters the name given to herbs that have a bitter taste. It may be due to a combination of chemicals within the plant. The herbs include angostura, yellow gentian, nux vomica and wormwood and they can be used as appetite stimulants, relaxant drugs and for their anti-inflammatory action.

carbohydrates these compounds are formed in plants as a result of photosynthesis. They include sugars, starches and cellulose which all have an important nutritional value. A polysaccharide is made up of hundreds of sugar molecules linked together, and they form part of compounds such as mucilage or pectin which help protect the alimentary canal. Carbohydrates are one of the main classes of naturally-derived organic compounds.

coumarins glycoside compounds widely distributed in plants. They provide the distinctive smell of many grass species.

ester organic compounds produced when an acid and an alcohol react. They often have distinctive fruity odours and are found naturally in fruits. An ester is generally a volatile liquid but may exist in a solid form.

fatty acids an organic compound made up of a hydrocarbon chain and a terminal carboxyl group (-COOH). The chain can range in length from one to thirty carbon atoms and branches can occur in the compound. Fatty acids are classified as saturated or unsaturated depending on the presence of a double bond in the chain structure. In nature, fatty acids form part of glycerides, that make up part of many important tissues and are important in many energy-releasing processes in the body.

flavonoid glycosides compounds made up of glycoside sugars and a flavone compound. The flavones are a group of chemicals, that give a yellow pigmentation to plants. This group of compounds is widely distributed through the plant kingdom, and they can have diuretic antispasmodic or stimulating effects on the body.

glucoside a term given to glycoside chemicals that contain glucose as the sugar.

glycoside molecules made up of two sections, a sugar and another chemical group. This name is given to all compounds independent of the sugar within them. As a class, glycosides are colourless, crystalline and bitter and are very common in plants. There are various classes of glycosides including cardiac glycosides, e.g. foxglove/digitalis and purgative glycosides, e.g. the anthraquinone chemicals in senna and rhubarb.

gum complex polysaccharides, that contain several different sugar and acid groups. They are generally soluble in water and produce viscous solutions, that are sometimes called mucilages. They are normally insoluble in organic solvents and are found in variable quantities in plant tissues.

hydrocarbons compounds made up of carbon and hydrogen alone. There are various categories of compounds, depending upon the arrangement of carbon atoms in the molecule and the number of double bonds in the molecule.

isomer compounds can have the same chemical composition and molecular weight but differ in their physical structure and hence are termed isomers. These isomers can have different physical and physiological qualities. Isomers can differ in the order in which the atoms are joined together (structural isomers) or they differ in the spatial orientation of atoms in the molecule (stereoisomerism). In plants, two isomeric forms of an active chemical may exist with one form having beneficial medical effects, and the other having no impact or a deleterious impact on the body. Care must be taken where several isomers of a chemical exist to utilize the correct form.

mucilage a gum-like substance found in the cell walls or seed coats of plants. They are polysaccharides that have a soothing effect on inflamed tissues, and they are used as an ingredient in some cosmetic preparations.

phenols slightly acidic compounds with at least one hydroxyl (-OH) group bonded to a carbon atom in an aromatic ring. They are widely found in natural plant constituents, e.g. tannins, anthocyanine glucoside pigments and salicylic acid. Salicylic acid frequently combines with a sugar to form a glycoside that has antiseptic properties, e.g. in crampbark, meadowsweet and white willow.

resin a naturally-produced acidic polymer obtained from trees. It is thought to help protect the tree from physical or mechanical damage, and attack by fungi and insects, in a similar way to how gums or mucilage protect green plants. It is a high molecular weight class of compounds usually produced by coniferous trees.

saponins glycosides that form a lather when shaken with water. They are found in two groups; the steroidal saponins that mimic the precursors of female sex hormones and the tri-terpenoid saponins that mimic the adrenocorticotropic hormone ACTH. They occur in a wide variety of plant groups and also act as a poison affecting fish.

starch a complex polysaccharide carbohydrate made by green plants during photosynthesis and which forms one of the plants' main energy stores. It is composed of water-soluble amylose and amylopectin, which forms a mucilaginous paste in water. Starch grains formed in the plant vary in size and shape according to the plant that produced them. Starch is used in industry as a food thickener, an adhesive and for sizing paper and cloth.

sugars a group of water-soluble carbohydrates with a sweet taste.

They can contain six or twelve carbon units in each molecule and the simple sugar units or monosaccharides can combine to form more complex sugar groups. It is a crystalline substance, found in many forms in plants.

tannins a group of complex organic chemicals found in the leaves, unripe fruits and bark of trees. They generally taste astringent and may be a protective mechanism against the grazing of some animals. They have commercial uses in treating cattle hides to produce leather, in producing ink and as mordants in the textile industry.

terpenes a group of unsaturated hydrocarbons, made up of multiples of isoprene units. The group includes vitamins A, E and K, carotene and other carotenoid pigments and squalene, the precursor to cholesterol. The terpenes are of great scientific and industrial importance. They are very reactive chemicals, with characteristic and pleasant odours that are used in perfumery.

volatile oil these compounds are formed from an alcohol and a hydrocarbon. They are found in many plants and can give a plant a characteristic taste and flavour. Many volatile oils have medicinal properties and are used as antifungal, antiseptic or aromatic oils taken internally or externally. They are very important oils in herbal medicine.

waxes fatty acid esters of alcohols with a high molecular weight. They are normally solid and have water-repellent properties. Waxes form a protective coating on animal skin, fur or feathers and also reduce water loss in leaves and fruits. The waxes are used for various commercial uses including polishes, textiles and pharmaceuticals.

Medical Glossary

amenorrhoea an absence of menstruation which is normal before puberty, during pregnancy and while breast-feeding is being carried out and following the menopause. Primary amenorrhoea describes the situation where the menstrual periods do not begin at puberty. This occurs if there is a chromosome abnormality (such as Turner's syndrome) or if some reproductive organs are absent. It can also occur where there is a failure or imbalance in the secretion of hormones. In secondary amenorrhoea, the menstrual periods stop when they would normally be expected to be present. There are a variety of causes including hormone deficiency, disorders of the hypothalamus, psychological and environmental stresses, during starvation, anorexia nervosa or depression.

arthritis inflammation of the joints or spine, the symptoms of which are pain and swelling, restriction of movement, redness and warmth of the skin. There are many different causes of arthritis including osteoarthritis, rheumatoid arthritis, tuberculosis and rheumatic fever.

asthma a condition characterized by breathing difficulties caused by narrowing of the airways (bronchi) of the lung. It is a distressing condition with breathlessness and a paroxysmal wheezing cough and the extent to which the bronchi narrow varies considerably. Asthma may occur at any age but usually begins in early childhood, and is a hypersensitive response that can be brought on by exposure to a variety of allergens, exercise, stress or infections. An asthma sufferer may have other hypersensitive conditions such as eczema and hay fever, and it may be prevalent within a family. It may or may not be possible for a person to avoid the allergen(s) responsible for an asthma attack. Treatment involves the use of drugs to dilate the airways (bronchodilators) and also inhaled corticosteroids.

atheroma a degenerative condition of the arteries. The inner and middle coats of the arterial walls become scarred and fatty deposits (cholesterol) are built up at these sites. The blood circulation is impaired and it may lead to such problems as angina pectoris, stroke and heart attack. The condition is associated with the western lifestyle. i.e. lack of exercise, smoking, obesity and too high an intake of animal fats.

atrophy wasting of a body part due to lack of use, malnutrition or as a result of ageing. The ovaries of women atrophy after the menopause and muscular atrophy accompanies certain diseases.

boil (or furuncle) a skin infection in a hair follicle or gland that produces inflammation and pus. The infection is often due to the bacterium *Staphylococcus*, but healing is generally quick upon release of the pus or administration of antibiotics. Frequent occurrence of boils is usually investigated to ensure the patient is not suffering from diabetes mellitus.

bronchitis occurring in two forms, acute and chronic, bronchitis is the inflammation of the bronchi. Bacteria or viruses cause the acute form that is typified by the symptoms of the common cold initially, but develops with painful coughing, wheezing, throat and chest pains and the production of purulent (pus-containing) mucus. If the infection spreads to the bronchioles (bronchiolitis) the consequences are even more serious as the body is deprived of oxygen. Antibiotics and expectorants can relieve the symptoms.

Chronic bronchitis is identified by an excessive production of mucus and may be due to recurrence of the acute form. It is a common cause of death among the elderly and there are several parameters of direct consequence to its cause: excessive smoking of cigarettes; cold, damp climate; obesity; respiratory infections. Damage to the bronchi and other complications may occur giving rise to constant breathlessness. Bronchodilator drugs are ineffective in treatment of the chronic form.

bruises injuries of, and leakage of blood into, the subcutaneous tissues, but without an open wound. In the simplest case minute vessels rupture and blood occupies the skin in the immediate area. A larger injury may be accompanied by swelling. A bruise begins as blue/black in colour, followed by brown and yellow as the blood pigment is reabsorbed.

burns burns and scalds show similar symptoms and require similar treatment, the former being caused by dry heat, the latter moist heat. Burns may also be due to electric currents and chemicals. Formerly burns were categorized by degrees (a system developed by Dupuytres, a French surgeon) but are now either superficial, where sufficient tissue remains to ensure skin regrows, or deep where grafting will be necessary.

Severe injuries can prove dangerous because of shock due to fluid loss at the burn. For minor burns and scalds, treatment involves holding the affected area under cold water. In more severe cases antiseptic dressings are normally applied and in very severe cases hospitalization is required. Morphine is usually administered to combat the pain. If the burns exceed nine per cent then a transfusion is required.

calculus stones formed within the body, particularly in the urinary tract (gravel) or gall bladder (see gallstones). They are formed from mineral salts, e.g. calcium oxalate and they generally cause pain as they may block the ureter or bile ducts. Treatment is by removing or crushing the stone surgically, by drugs and diet (in gallstones a low fat diet eases pain and prevents formation of more stones) and also by the use of herbal remedies.

cancer a widely-used term describing any form of malignant tumour. Characteristically, there is an uncontrolled and abnormal growth of cancer cells that invade surrounding tissues and destroy them. Cancer cells may spread throughout the body via the blood stream or lymphatic system, a process known as metastasis, and set up secondary growths elsewhere. There are known to be a number of different causes of cancer including cigarette smoking, radiation, ultraviolet light, some viruses and possibly the presence of cancer genes (oncogenes). Treatment depends upon the site of the cancer but involves radiotherapy, chemotherapy and surgery, and survival rates in affected people are showing encouraging improvements.

chilblain a round, itchy inflammation of the skin that usually occurs on the toes or fingers during cold weather, and is caused by a localized deficiency in the circulation. Chilblains may sometimes be an indication of poor health or inadequate clothing and nutrition. Keeping the feet and hands warm, paying attention to the diet and exercise to improve the circulation help to prevent chilblains.

cholera an infection of the small intestine caused by the bacterium *Vibrio cholerae*. It varies in degree from very mild cases to extremely severe illness and death. The disease originated in Asia but spread widely last century when there were great cholera epidemics in Britain and elsewhere. During epidemics of cholera, the death rate is over fifty per cent and these occur in conditions of poor sanitation and overcrowding. The disease is spread through contamination of drinking water by faeces of those affected by the disease, and also by flies landing on infected material and then crawling on food.

Epidemics are rare in conditions of good sanitation but when cholera is detected, extreme attention has to be paid to hygiene including treatment and scrupulous disposal of the body waste of the infected person. The incubation period for cholera is one to five days and then a person suffers from severe vomiting and diarrhoea (known as "cholera diarrhoea" or "rice water stools"). This results in severe dehydration and death may follow within twenty four hours. Treatment involves bed rest and the taking by mouth of salt solutions, or these may need to be given intravenously.Tetracycline or other sulphonamide drugs are given to kill the bacteria. The death rate is low (five per cent) in those given proper and prompt treatment but the risk is greater in children and the elderly. Vaccination against cholera can be given but it is only effective for about six months.

chorea a disorder of the nervous system characterized by the involuntary, jerky movements of the muscles mainly of the face, shoulders and hips. *Sydenham's chorea* or *St. Vitus' dance* is a disease that mainly affects children and is associated with acute rheumatism. About one third of affected children develop rheumatism elsewhere in the body, often involving the heart, and the disease is more common in girls than in boys. If the heart is affected there may be problems in later life but treatment consists of rest and the giving of mild sedatives. The condition usually recovers over a period of a few months. *Huntington's chorea* is an inherited condition that does not appear until after the age of forty and is accompanied by dementia. *Senile chorea* afflicts some elderly people but there is no dementia.

cirrhosis a disease of the liver in which fibrous tissue resembling scar tissue is produced as a result of damage and death to the cells. The liver becomes yellow-coloured and nodular in appearance, and there are various types of the disease including alcoholic cirrhosis and postnecrotic cirrhosis caused by viral hepatitis. The cause of the cirrhosis is not always found (cryptogenic cirrhosis) but the progress of the condition can be halted if this can be identified and removed. This particularly is applicable in alcoholic cirrhosis where the consumption of alcohol has to cease.

cold (common cold) widespread and mild infection of the upper respiratory tract caused by a virus. There is inflammation of the mucous membranes and symptoms include feverishness, coughing, sneezing, runny nose, sore throat, headache and sometimes face ache due to catarrh in the sinuses. The disease is spread by coughing and sneezing and treatment is by means of bed rest and the taking of mild analgesics.

conjunctivitis inflammation of the mucous membrane (conjunctiva) that lines the inside of the eyelid and covers the front of the eye. The eyes become pink and watery and the condition is usually caused by an infection that may be bacterial, viral or the microorganism *Chlamydia* may be responsible. Treatment depends upon cause but a number of drugs are used often in the form of eyedrops.

constipation the condition in which the bowels are opened too infrequently and the faeces become dry, hard and difficult and painful to pass. The frequency of normal bowel opening varies between people but when constipation becomes a problem, it is usually a result of inattention to this habit or to the diet. To correct the condition a change of lifestyle may be needed including taking more exercise, fluid and roughage in the diet. Laxatives and enemas are also used to alleviate the condition. Constipation is also a symptom of the more serious condition of blockage of the bowel (by a tumour), but this is less common.

convulsions also known as fits, these are involuntary, alternate, rapid, muscular contractions and relaxations throwing the body and limbs into contortions. They are caused by a disturbance of brain function and in adults usually result from epilepsy. In babies and young children they occur quite commonly but, although alarming, are generally not serious. Causes include a high fever due to infection, brain diseases such as meningitis and breath-holding, that is quite common in infants and very young children. Convulsions are thought to be more common in the very young because the nervous system is immature. Unless they are caused by the presence of disease or infection that requires to be treated, they are rarely life-threatening.

cramp prolonged and painful spasmodic muscular contraction that often occurs in the limbs but can affect certain internal organs. Cramp may result from a salt imbalance as in heat cramp. Working in high temperatures causes excessive sweating and consequent loss of salt. It can be corrected and prevented by an increase of the salt intake. Occupational cramp results from continual repetitive use of particular muscles, e.g. writer's cramp. Night cramp occurs during sleep and is especially common among elderly people, diabetics and pregnant women. The cause is not known.

croup a group of diseases characterized by a swelling, partial obstruction and inflammation of the entrance to the larynx, occurring in young children. The breathing is harsh and strained producing a typical crowing sound, accompanied by coughing and feverishness. Diphtheria used to be the most common cause of croup but it now usually results from a viral infection of the respiratory tract (laryngo-tracheo bronchitis). The condition is relieved by inhaling steam and also by mild sedatives and/or pain killers. Rarely, the obstruction becomes dangerous and completely blocks the larynx in which case emergency tracheostomy or nasotracheal intubation may be required. Usually, the symptoms of croup subside and the child recovers, but then he or she may have a tendency towards attacks on future occasions.

delirium a mental disorder typified by confusion, agitation, fear, anxiety, illusions and sometimes hallucinations. The causal cerebral disfunction may be due to deficient nutrition, stress, toxic poisoning or mental shock.

depression a mental state of extreme sadness dominated by pessimism and in which normal behaviour patterns (sleep, appetite, etc.) are disturbed. Causes are varied upsetting events, loss, etc. and treatment involves the use of therapy and drugs.

diarrhoea increased frequency and looseness of bowel movement, involving the passage of unusually soft faeces. Diarrhoea can be caused by food poisoning, colitis, irritable bowel syndrome, dysentery, etc. A severe case will result in the loss of water and salts that must be replaced and anti-diarrhoeal drugs are used in certain circumstances.

diphtheria a serious, infectious disease caused by the bacterium *Corynebacterium diphtheriae,* and commonest in children. The infection causes a membranous lining on the throat that can interfere with breathing and eating. The toxin produced by the bacterium damages heart tissue and the central nervous system and it can be fatal if not treated. The infection is countered by injection of the antitoxin with penicillin or erythromycin taken to kill the bacterium. Diphtheria can be immunized against.

dropsy old-fashioned name for oedema.

dysentery an infection and ulceration of the lower part of the bowels that causes severe diarrhoea with the passage of mucus and blood. There are two forms of dysentery caused by different organisms. Amoebic dysentery is due to *Entamoeba histolytica* that is spread via infected food or water and occurs mainly in the tropics and sub-tropics. The appearance of symptoms may be delayed but in addition to diarrhoea there is indigestion, anaemia and weight loss. Drugs are used in treatment.

Bacillary dysentery is caused by the bacterium *Shigella* and spreads by contact with a carrier or contaminated food. Symptoms appear from one to six days after infection and include diarrhoea, cramp, nausea, fever and the severity of the attack varies. Antibiotics may be given to kill the bacteria but recovery usually occurs within one to two weeks.

dysmenorrhoea painful menstruation. There are two main types, primary and secondary. Primary or spasmodic dysmenorrhoea is extremely common, but is normally mild and short-lived in duration. In a small proportion of women, the pain is severe enough to cause partial or total debility. The pain generally occurs in the lower abdomen or back and is cramping, often coming in waves that is due to uterine contractions. It is associated with dizziness, nausea, vomiting, headache, fainting and pale complexion with obvious distress. Secondary or congestive dysmenorrhoea is pain with a congested ache and cramps in the lower abdomen. It is generally due to specific pelvic conditions, e.g. chronic pelvic infection, endometriosis, fibroid tumours and the presence of an interuterine contraceptive device (IUCD).

eczema an inflammation of the skin that causes itching, a red rash and often small blisters that weep and become encrusted. This may be followed by the skin thickening and then peeling off in scales. There are several types of eczema, *atopic* being one of the most common. (Atopic is the hereditary tendency to form allergic reactions due to an antibody in the skin). A form of atopic eczema is infantile eczema that starts at three or four months and it is often the case that eczema, hay fever and asthma is found in the family history. However, many children improve markedly as they approach the age of ten or eleven. The treatment for such conditions usually involves the use of hydrocortisone and other steroid creams and ointments.

epilepsy a neurological disorder involving convulsions, seizures and loss of consciousness. There are many possible causes or associations of epilepsy, including cerebral trauma, brain tumour, cerebral haemorrhage and metabolic imbalances as in hypoglycaemia. Usually an epileptic attack occurs without warning, with complete unconsciousness and some muscle contraction and spasms. Some drugs are used in treatment although little can be done during the fit itself.

erysipelas an infectious disease, caused by *Streptococcus pyogenes*. It produces an inflammation of the skin with associated redness. Large areas of the body may be affected and other symptoms may include vesicles, fever and pain with a feeling of heat and a tingling sensation. In addition to being isolated, patients are given penicillin.

fistula an abnormal opening between two hollow organs or between such an organ or gland and the exterior. These may arise during development so that a baby may be born with a fistula. Alternatively, they can be produced by injury, infection or as a complication following surgery. A common example is an anal fistula, that may develop if an abscess present in the rectum bursts and produces a communication through the surface of the skin. An operation is normally required to correct a fistula, but healing is further complicated in the case of an anal fistula because of the passage of waste material through the bowels.

gallstones stones of varying composition, that form in the gall bladder. Their formation seems to be due to a change in bile composition rendering cholesterol less soluble. Stones may also form around a foreign body. There are three types of stone cholesterol, pigment and mixed, the latter being the most common. Calcium salts are usually found in varying proportions. Although gallstones may be present for years without symptoms, they can cause severe pain and may pass into the common bile duct to cause, by the resulting obstruction, jaundice.

gleet discharge due to chronic gonorrhoea.

gonorrhoea the most common venereal disease that is spread primarily by sexual intercourse but may be contracted through contact with infected discharge on clothing, towels, etc. The causative agent is the bacterium *Neisseria gonorrhoeae* and it affects the mucous membrane of the vagina, or in the male, the urethra. Symptoms develop approximately one week after infection and include pain on urinating with a discharge of pus. Inflammation of nearby organs may occur (testicle, prostate in men; uterus, Fallopian tubes and ovaries in women) and prolonged inflammation of the urethra may lead to formation of fibrous tissue causing stricture. Joints may also be affected and later complications include endocarditis, arthritis and conjunctivitis.

If a baby is born to a woman with the disease, the baby's eyes may become infected, until recently a major cause of blindness (called *Ophthalmia neonatorum*). Treatment is usually very effective through the administration of penicillin, sulphonamides or tetracycline.

gout a disorder caused by an imbalance of uric acid in the body. Uric acid is normally excreted by the kidneys but sufferers of gout have an excess in their bloodstream that is deposited in joints as salts (urates) of the acid. This causes inflammation of the affected joints and painful gouty arthritis with destruction of the joints. The kidneys may also be damaged, with formation of stones. Deposits of the salts (called *tophi*) may reach the stage where they prohibit further use of the joints, causing hands and feet to be set in a particular position. Treatment of gout is through drugs that increase the excretion of the urate salts or slow their formation.

gravel this name refers to small stones formed in the urinary tract. They normally are made up of calcareous material and crystalline matter and passage of stones from the kidneys is normally linked to severe pain and, possibly, the presence of blood in the urine.

haemorrhoids (piles) varicose and inflamed veins around the lower end of the bowel situated in the wall of the anus. They are classified as internal, external and mixed depending upon whether they appear beyond the anus. They are commonly caused by constipation or diarrhoea, especially in middle and older age, and may be exacerbated by a sedentary life style. They may also occur as a result of childbearing. Symptoms of haemorrhoids are bleeding and pain, and treatment is by means of creams, injections and suppositories. Attention to diet (to treat constipation) and regular exercise are important, but in severe cases, surgery to remove the haemorrhoids may be necessary.

hysteria a type of neurosis that is difficult to define and in which a range of symptoms may occur. These include paralysis, seizures and spasms of limbs, swelling of joints, mental disorders and amnesia. The person is vulnerable to suggestion. Two types are recognized, *conversion hysteria* that is characterized by physical symptoms and *dissociative hysteria* in which marked mental changes occur. *Mass hysteria* affects a group, especially those gathered together under conditions of emotional excitement. A number of people may suffer from giddiness, vomiting and fainting that runs through the whole crowd. Recovery occurs when those affected are separated from the others under calmer conditions. Treatment for hysteria is by means of psychotherapy, involving suggestion.

influenza a highly infectious disease caused by a virus that affects the respiratory tract. Symptoms include headache, weakness and fever, appetite loss and general aches and pains. Sometimes there is the complication of a lung infection that requires immediate treatment. There are three main strains of influenza virus, designated A, B and C. The viruses quickly produce new strains which is why an attack of one is unlikely to provide protection against a later bout of the disease. Epidemics occur periodically and in Britain virus A is responsible for the majority of outbreaks.

jaundice a condition characterized by the unusual presence of bile pigment (bilirubin) in the blood. The bile produced in the liver passes into the blood instead of the intestines and because of this there is a yellowing of the skin and the whites of the eyes.

There are several types of jaundice: *obstructive* due to bile not reaching the intestine due to an obstruction e.g. a gallstone; *haemolytic* where red blood cells are destroyed by haemolysis; *hepatocellular* due to a liver disease such as hepatitis which results in the liver being unable to use the bilirubin. *Neonatal jaundice* is quite common in newborn infants when the liver is physiologically immature but it usually lasts only a few days. The infant can be exposed to blue light that converts bilirubin to biliverdin, another (harmless) bile pigment.

laryngitis inflammation of the mucous membrane that lines the larynx and vocal cords. It is due to viral infection in the main, but also bacteria, chemical irritants, heavy smoking or excessive use of the voice. *Acute* laryngitis accompanies infections of the upper respiratory tract and the symptoms include pain, a cough, difficulty in swallowing. *Chronic* laryngitis may be due to recurrence of the acute form, but is often attributable to excessive smoking worsened by alcohol. Changes occurring in the vocal cords are more permanent and the symptoms are as for the acute form, but longer lasting.

leucorrhea a discharge of white or yellow-coloured mucus from the vagina. It may be a normal condition, increasing before and after menstruation but a large discharge probably indicates an infection somewhere in the genital tract. A common cause is the infection called thrush but it may also be due to gonorrhoea in which case the treatment will differ.

malaria an infectious disease caused by the presence of minute parasitic organisms of the genus *Plasmodium* in the blood. The disease is characterized by recurrent bouts of fever and anaemia, the interval between the attacks depending upon the species. The parasite is transmitted to man by the *Anopheles* mosquito, (common in sub-tropical and tropical regions) being present in the salivary glands and passed into the bloodstream of a person when the insect bites. Similarly, the parasite is ingested by the mosquito when it takes a blood meal from an infected person. Efforts to control malaria have centred on destruction of the mosquito and its breeding sites. Once injected into the blood, the organisms concentrate in the liver where they multiply and then re-enter the bloodstream destroying red blood cells. This releases the parasites causing shivering, fever, sweating and anaemia. The process is then repeated, with hours or days between attacks. Drugs are used both to prevent infection, although these may not be totally effective, and to cure the disease once present.

nephritis inflammation of the kidney, that may be due to one of several causes. Types of nephritis include glomerulonephritis (when the glomerulus is affected), acute nephritis, hereditary nephritis, etc.

neuralgia strictly, pain in some part or the whole of a nerve (without any physical change in the nerve) but used more widely to encompass pain following the course of a nerve or its branches, whatever the cause. Neuralgia often occurs at the same time each day and is frequently an agonizing pain. It occurs in several forms and is named accordingly, e.g. sciatica, trigeminal neuralgia (affecting the face) and intercostal neuralgia (affecting the ribs). Treatment often involves the application of ointments, and the taking of pain-killing drugs. If such treatments do not bring relief, it is possible to freeze the nerve or destroy part of it by surgery.

oedema an accumulation of fluid in the body, possibly beneath the skin or in cavities or organs. With an injury the swelling may be localized or more general as in cases of kidney or heart failure. Fluid can collect in the chest cavity, abdomen or lung (pulmonary oedema). The causes are numerous, e.g. cirrhosis of the liver, heart or kidney failure, starvation, acute nephritis, allergies or drugs. To alleviate the symptom, the root cause has to be removed. Subcutaneous oedema commonly occurs in women before menstruation, as swollen legs or ankles, but does subside if the legs are rested in a raised position.

palsy the term used formerly for paralysis and retained for the names of some conditions.

pleurisy (*or* **pleuritis**) inflammation of the pleura resulting in pain from deep breathing, and resulting shortness of breath. There is a typical frictional rub heard through a stethoscope. Pleurisy is often due to pneumonia in the adjacent lung and is always associated with disease in the lung, diaphragm, chest wall or abdomen e.g. tuberculosis, abscesses, bronchial carcinoma, etc.

pneumonia a bacterial infection of the lungs resulting in inflammation and filling of the alveoli with pus and fluid. As a result the lung becomes solid and air cannot enter. The symptoms vary depending upon how much of the lung is unavailable for respiration, but commonly there will be chest pain, coughing, breathlessness, fever and possibly cyanosis. Pneumonia may be caused by several bacteria, viruses or fungi, but bacterial infection is commonest. Bronchopneumonia affects the bronchi and bronchioles; lobar pneumonia the whole lobes of the lung(s). Antibiotic treatment is usually effective although it helps to know which is the infecting organism, to provide the most specific treatment.

prolapse a moving down of an organ or tissue from its normal position due to the supporting tissues weakening. This may happen to the lower end of the bowel (in children) or the uterus and vagina in women who have sustained some sort of injury during childbirth. In the latter case prolapse may result in the uterus itself showing on the outside. Surgery can shorten the supporting ligaments and narrow the vaginal opening.

psoriasis a chronic skin disease for which the cause is unknown and the treatment is palliative. The affected skin appears as itchy, scaly red areas, starting usually around the elbows and knees. It often runs in families and may be associated with anxiety, commencing usually in childhood or adolescence. Treatment involves the use of ointments and creams.

rheumatism a general term used to describe aches and pains in joints and muscles.

rickets a disease affecting children that involves a deficiency of vitamin D. Vitamin D can be manufactured in the skin in the presence of sunlight but dietary sources are important especially where sunlight is lacking. The disease is characterized by soft bones that bend out of shape and cause deformities.

Bones are hardened by the deposition of calcium salts and

this cannot happen in the absence of vitamin D. Treatment consists of giving vitamin D, usually in the form of calciferol, and ensuring that there is an adequate amount in the child's future diet. Vitamin D deficiency in adults causes the condition called osteomalacia.

scarlet fever an infectious disease, mainly of childhood, caused by the bacterium *Streptococcus*. Symptoms show after a few days and include sickness, sore throat, fever and a scarlet rash that may be widespread. Antibiotics are effective and also prevent any complications e.g. inflammation of the kidneys.

sciatica pain in the sciatic nerve, and therefore felt in the back of the thigh, leg and foot. The commonest cause is a prolapsed intervertebral disc pressing on a nerve root, but it may also be due to ankylosing spondylitis and other conditions.

scurvy a deficiency disease caused by a lack of vitamin C (ascorbic acid) due to a dietary lack of fruit and vegetables. Symptoms begin with swollen, bleeding gums and then subcutaneous bleeding, bleeding into joints, ulcers, anaemia and then fainting, diarrhoea and trouble with major organs. Untreated, it is fatal, but nowadays it is easily prevented, or cured should it arise, through correct diet or administration of the vitamin.

smallpox a highly infectious viral disease that has nonetheless been eradicated. Infection results, after about two weeks, in a high fever, head and body aches and vomiting. Eventually red spots appear that change to water and then pus-filled vesicles that on drying out leave scars. The person stays infectious until all scabs are shed. Fever often returns, with delirium. Recovery is usual, but complications often ensue, e.g. pneumonia. The last naturally-occurring case was in 1977.

stone another name for calculus.

strangury the desire to pass water, that can only be done in a few drops and with accompanying pain. It is symptomatic of an irritation of the base of the bladder by a stone, cancer at this site, or cystitis or prostatitis.

syphilis an infectious, sexually-transmitted disease, caused by the bacterium *Treponema pallidum* that shows symptoms in three stages. Bacteria enter the body through mucous membranes during sexual intercourse and an ulcer appears in the first instance. Within a short time the lymph nodes locally and then all over the body enlarge and harden and this lasts several weeks.

Secondary symptoms appear about two months after infection and include fever, pains, enlarged lymph nodes and a faint rash that is usually noticed on the chest. The bacterium is found in enormous numbers in the primary sores and any skin lesions of the secondary stage. The final stage may not appear until many months or years after infection and comprises the formation of numerous tumour-like masses throughout the body (in skin, muscle, bone, brain, spinal cord and other organs such as the liver, stomach, etc.). This stage can cause serious damage to the heart, brain or spinal cod resulting in blindness, tabes dorsalis, and mental disability.

Congenital syphilis is much rarer than the former, *acquired*, type. It is contracted by a developing foetus from the mother, across the placenta and symptoms show a few weeks after birth. Treatment of syphilis is with penicillin, but it should be administered early in the development of the disease.

torpor a state of physical and mental sluggishness that accompanies various mental disorders, some kinds of poisoning and may be present in elderly people with arterial disease.

tuberculosis a group of infections caused by the bacillus (bacterium) *Mycobacterium tuberculosis* of which pulmonary tuberculosis of the lungs (consumption or phthisis) is the best known form. The pulmonary disease is acquired through inhalation of air containing the organism from an infected person, or dust laden with bacteria. People infected in this way can show no symptoms but still be carriers. In the lungs, the infection causes formation of a *primary tubercle* that spreads to lymph nodes to form the *primary complex*.

The disease may wax and wane for years as the body's natural immune system acts against the infection. If the infection is severe, symptoms include fever, wasting, night sweats and the coughing up of blood. The bacteria may enter the blood stream and spread throughout the body setting up numerous tubercles in other tissues (*Miliary tuberculosis*). The organism may also be acquired by eating contaminated food, especially milk, in which case the production of a primary complex in abdominal lymph nodes can lead to peritonitis. Rarely, the infection is acquired via a cut from contact with an infected person or animal. Tuberculosis affects people throughout the world (about six thousand new cases each year in England and Wales). Many people acquire the infection and recover without suspecting its presence and the disease is curable with antibiotics, e.g. streptomycin. In addition, BCG vaccination as a preventive measure is given to children in the U.K., in addition to X-ray screening to detect carriers.

ulcer a break on the skin surface or on the mucous membrane lining within the body cavities that may be inflamed and fails to heal. Ulcers of the skin include bedsores and varicose ulcers (that are caused by defective circulation). Ulcers of the alimentary tract include duodenal ulcers, gastric ulcers and peptic ulcers.

varicose veins that have become stretched, distended and twisted. The superficial veins in the legs are often affected although it may occur elsewhere. Causes include congenitally defective valves, obesity, pregnancy and also thrombophlebitis (inflammation of the wall of a vein with secondary thrombosis in the affected part of the vein). Elastic support is a common treatment although alternatives are sclerotherapy and phlebectomy.

whooping cough (*pertussis*) an infectious disease caused by the bacterium *Bordetella pertussis*. The mucous membranes lining the air passages are affected and after a one to two week incubation period, fever, catarrh and a cough develop. The cough then becomes paroxysmal with a number of short coughs punctuated with the 'whooping' drawing in of breath. Nosebleeds and vomiting may follow a paroxysm. After about two weeks the symptoms abate but a cough may continue for some weeks. Whooping cough is not usually serious and immunization reduces the severity of an attack. However, a child may be susceptible to pneumonia and tuberculosis during the disease.